SPIRITUALLY FLY

SPIRITUALLY FLY

WISDOM, MEDITATIONS, AND YOGA
TO ELEVATE YOUR SOUL

FAITH HUNTER

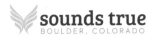
sounds true
BOULDER, COLORADO

Sounds True
Boulder, CO 80306

This book is not intended as a substitute for the medical recommendations of
physicians, mental health professionals, or other health-care providers. Rather, it is
intended to offer information to help the reader cooperate with physicians, mental
health professionals, and health-care providers in a mutual quest for optimal well-
being. We advise readers to carefully review and understand the ideas presented
and to seek the advice of a qualified professional before attempting to use them.

Published 2021

Cover design by Rachael Murray
Book design by Karen Polaski

Cover and interior photographs © Brooks Freehill

Printed in South Korea

BK05839

Library of Congress Cataloging-in-Publication Data
Names: Hunter, Faith (Yoga and Meditation Instructor), author.
Title: Spiritually fly : wisdom, meditations, and yoga to elevate your soul / Faith Hunter.
Description: Boulder, CO: Sounds True, 2021.
Identifiers: LCCN 2020038183 (print) | LCCN 2020038184 (ebook) |
    ISBN 9781683643753 (paperback) | ISBN 9781683644262 (ebook)
Subjects: LCSH: Yoga. | Spiritual life.
Classification: LCC B132.Y6 H86 2021 (print) | LCC
    B132.Y6 (ebook) | DDC 204/.36—dc23
LC record available at https://lccn.loc.gov/2020038183
LC ebook record available at https://lccn.loc.gov/2020038184

10 9 8 7 6 5 4 3 2 1

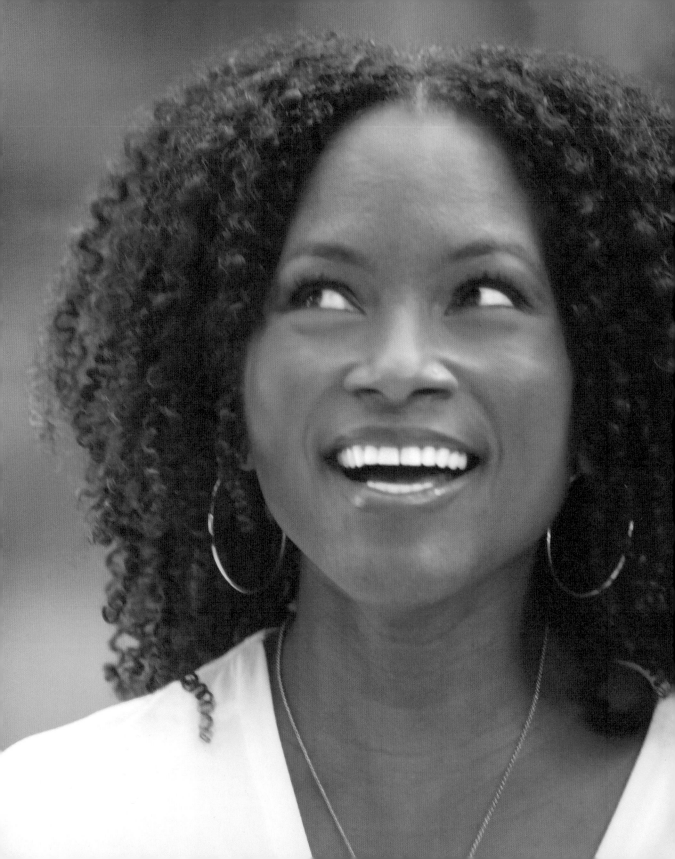

For Mother, Dad,
Mark, and Michael:
my soul is your soul.

To my 5-year old self:
I finally see you!

CONTENTS

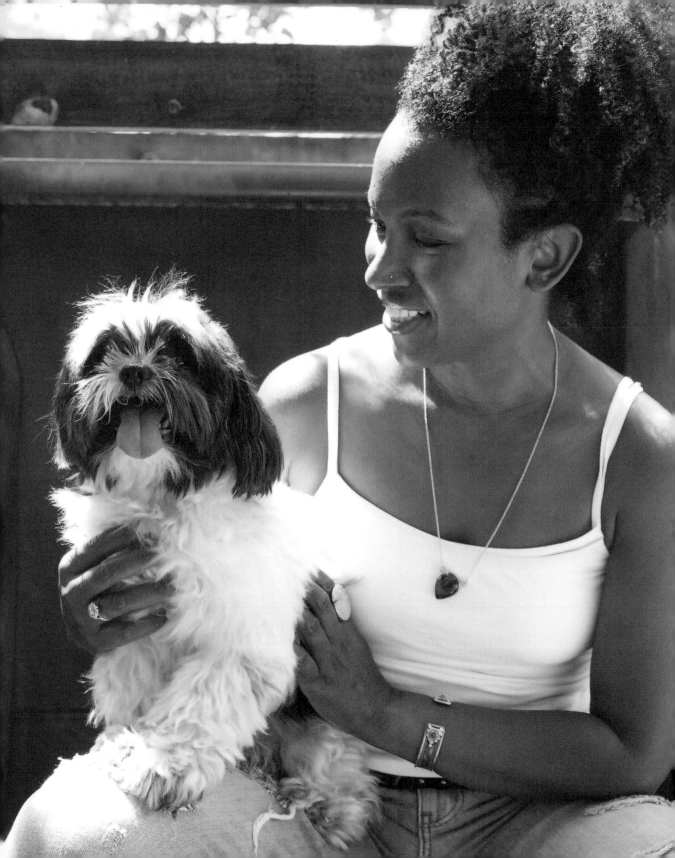

INTRODUCTION

your path to flyness

god, where are you? This is Faith, and I need you now. I need you to free me from the angst, discomfort, and overall bad luck. Screaming uncontrollably, I'm falling to my knees, and begging for mercy. If you don't answer, I'm walking away, and cursing your name. I'm done with the play on my emotions. I'm sick of you delivering a moment of joy, and then months later, you snatching it all away. I second-guess myself on every decision, and regardless of failure or success, I regret the direction I decided on. I'm also exhausted by guilty feelings around spirituality and fearful of what excruciating experience is around the corner as a believer or not. Seriously, God, I've been a good girl, praised your name, and still, horrible things have happened. The pain, shame, and suffering has paralyzed my mind and tainted my heart. I'm standing here naked, womb exposed, belly rotating, and spiraling into darkness with the hope of you grabbing my hand. Please help. I can't do this any longer.

This was my internal testimonial for many years. As a young black girl growing up in rural Louisiana, I spent most of my childhood steeped in the doctrine of the Baptist church. God was my lord and savior, and this was where I found strength. Even to this day, I can easily recite the Lord's Prayer on command. As I write this paragraph, the prayer is racing through my mind, flecked with memories of the New Rocky Valley Baptist Church. I hear the choir, I see myself wearing a white gown, and I recall the pastor telling me to walk into the water. I was ten years old, getting baptized and committing myself to God. There was nothing more divine than to feel I was saved through glorified ritual, but little did I know that it would take more than a dip in "holy water" to free me from sin.

WE ARE ALL DIVINE BEINGS WALKING A PATH

In the 1980s, I struggled daily as a young girl to find the answers and salvation within biblical text. I regularly flipped through the Bible for God's guidance on such matters as the Mount St. Helens volcano eruption and the divorce of my classmates' parents. Multiple times per week I would open my little green King James Bible and just read. The more I experienced in life, the more I would read and attempt to understand. I even found myself drifting off during Sunday school wondering why God talked to my grandparents but never answered my questions or prayers. My greatest question revolved around why my brothers were infected with HIV. I simply couldn't figure out why, if God was real, he didn't stop this from happening. As a result, I drifted into my twenties with a lack of divine alignment or spiritual connection. While my outer layer was glittered with southern charm and perfect manners, my inner self was a hot mess.

At the age of twenty-three, while my older brother was fighting for his life, I rolled into my first yoga class. It was the 1990s and an interesting time in my life, but it was hard for me to focus on anything but work, graduate school, beauty pageants, and a family in turmoil. The yoga experience was odd, but a dear friend thought it would help.

I recall doing a little yoga on PBS with Rodney Yee around the same time, but the yoga room surrounded by the noise of men dropping weights was nothing like Yee's Hawaiian practice. Wearing all white, the teacher opened with a chant I didn't understand, guided us through some type of deep breathing, and told us to "keep up or be kept up." Then somewhere between thinking "I'm strong" and collapsing in tears, I felt a spark. Within the spark appeared a moment of silence in my head. For a few breaths I didn't ponder the looming death of my brother, the arguments between my parents, or the fact that I probably needed to leave grad school for a semester. There was something about this yoga class that gave me a moment to be alone in a crowded gym.

Soon I realized I was practicing kundalini yoga. As I related to the physical intensity of the practice, the teacher created a safe space for my emotional breakdowns. The class literally became my weekly cry fest. I curled into forward bends and cried almost every time in final relaxation. With tiny bits of belief in my heart, I even prayed the purifying power of Breath of Fire would do the trick.

Soon elements of the class merged into my life. After a long day at work and evenings in the hospital visiting my brother, I would return home and meditate before bed. And somehow that one yoga class a week gave me hope. On yoga days I would wake up less depressed, rarely argued with my mother, and always felt excited to stop by the hospital to kiss my brother good night. Yoga didn't supply the answers, but it was enough to release a few layers of pain.

Throughout the late 1990s and into the 2000s, I diligently practiced yoga and meditation. At the same time, I battled with my belief in God and the self. Even when I found vinyasa yoga, there were moments in the flow of Sun Salutation that I thought of floating away from it all. I hated my life and thought God and all those religious teachings were a joke. I would hear yoga teachers talk about how lovely it was to be alive, and those talks would trigger the same crap I questioned as a girl.

By 2001 my brother had died, my father had been diagnosed with cancer, and I was on the verge of getting a divorce. There was nothing joyous about my life or the people in it. My self-pity was over the top, yet the paradoxes of my childhood spiritual beliefs were strong. I felt very disconnected from the teachings but still aligned with the scriptures. For instance, in the morning, I would read Psalm 143:8: "Let the morning bring me word of your unfailing love, for I have put my trust in you. Show me the way I should go, for to you I entrust my life," and I trusted that the upcoming day would be better and less painful than the day before. I would say to friends that I wasn't religious or spiritual, but I prayed before eating a meal. Oddly enough I remained attached to who I am, Faith Hunter.

THE PAST WILL SHED LIGHT ON THE FUTURE

In college, I had an amazing philosophy professor, Dr. Horton. It's strange how the universe works. I was a marketing major and was only required to take one philosophy class, but out of all my college professors, Dr. Horton was one of my favorites. He had a brilliant ability to relate philosophical principles to modern life, and he introduced me to the Yoga Sutras of Patanjali. As he creatively guided us through the 196 threads of spiritual awakening, I was drawn to the beauty of the text and the concept that I could actually experience bliss. One of the sutras I found most intriguing was 1.40. It referred to how we as humans have the capacity to control the mind and the ability to concentrate on the smallest atom or the vast universe. Within this purified mind, all is possible. As I struggled with my religious God, the Yoga Sutras opened a door to the belief that I was powerful in some way. Although I didn't reopen a copy of the Yoga Sutras until I enrolled in yoga-teacher training in 2003, I held on to the hope of experiencing spirit in some capacity.

On Thanksgiving in 2002, I unrolled my yoga mat on the left side of a tiny yoga studio on Christopher Street in New York City. I had walked into Laughing Lotus Yoga Center, and my heart chakra was doing a glittery dance. Prior to practicing in this space my yoga experiences were relatively low-key. Laughing Lotus filled the space with the witty laughter of people from all walks of life, and the teachers encouraged us to be ourselves while at the same time loudly playing Prince's "1999." The center had bright colors on all the walls, and there was a blend of personal devotion, real New York life, and mystical play on the mat. This became my home away from home, and it slowly opened my heart to spiritual exploration.

I eventually graduated in 2003 from their yoga-teacher training and after a few years of teaching yoga in New York City, I decided to live with my younger brother in Washington, DC. It was 2006, and so much had changed about the city since my days of working in nonprofit during the Clinton era. I returned to working in nonprofit, and I taught yoga at night in a local studio and at gyms. To my surprise, the DC yoga industry was nothing like it was in New York where I had worked full-time as a yoga teacher. In fact, the yoga scene in DC truly sucked. There was zero diversity, and students complained about my music and method of teaching.

Within a year, I opened a yoga studio—Shakti Mind Body—with another African American yoga teacher. We both disliked the energy and atmosphere of other studios in the city, so we created a more appealing environment, and our Mt. Vernon Triangle location soon became a haven for all types of people. But the highlight was that we were the first studio in the DMV (DC/Maryland/Virginia) area where people of color could be trained by people of color.

Unable to step away from my church roots, I taught a yoga class—my form of spirituality—every Sunday morning. Merged with my own flavor, it was joyous, challenging, and always had a message. One of our regulars, who was devoted to my Sunday morning class, arrived one day and explained that her Baptist minister was concerned that she wasn't attending Sunday morning service anymore. My mind projected a variety of negative thoughts that mostly related to the religious teaching that Sunday was reserved for worshiping God and that all good Christians go to church on Sunday. But I held my tongue and allowed to her shed light on the dilemma.

She was torn between yoga and church but wanted nothing more than to keep yoga as an integral part of her Sunday ritual. She asked my opinion, and I told her to listen to her soul. The following Sunday she returned, drifted quietly to her favorite spot, unrolled her pink yoga mat, and practiced her yoga. I later asked what she had decided to do. She responded, "Sunday morning yoga feels best on a spiritual level, and this is what I need to kick off my week. So I'll see my minister on Wednesday nights for Bible study." She went on to share that practicing on Sunday was the right amount of Holy Ghost infused with modern teachings and urban vibrations, and it was "spiritually fly."

The next day I woke up and decided to change the name of my Sunday class to Spiritually Fly. I wasn't sure why it needed to be this, but my student's experience reminded me that spirit lives within. The practice I had been sharing and the experience we were having was filled with our collective spirit. It wasn't saturated with religious dogma, but instead it blended ancient healing technologies with a modern application. Based on what students needed and what heart was speaking, the class was about being present, for at least ninety minutes, for your own soul. I found myself stepping outside of who I thought students wanted me to be and began to fully teach from my own experience. The class was a must in the lives of my students, and their presence and authenticity became a benevolent offering in my life. Since 2007, my Sunday class has morphed into workshops and a lifestyle, and it is now my spiritual practice.

THE BIRTH OF THE SPIRITUALLY FLY SUTRAS

In 2011, I went through a traumatic personal relationship filled with control and abuse at the hands of my fiancé. It was a very confusing time because it returned me to a place of asking, why me? It made me wonder if I was truly causing the problems, or maybe God was cursing me after a period of good times. The relationship and my spiritual quandary thrust me into intense personal work, which resulted in the birth of the Spiritually Fly sutras. These sutras are my foundation, my breath, and my holy connection to spirit! Birthing the sutras involved more than yoga and meditation. It included a variety of tools that somehow pulled me out of the muck. I retreated into a personal cave of yoga, meditation, and self-reflection, and while many late nights in my apartment were flooded with conflicted thoughts, anger, sadness, and discomfort, I was able to reexamine my life without judgment. The healing and self-love tonics were emotionally draining, yet spiritually awakening.

I realized that I needed to pull together the best of everything I knew and had been teaching into a daily personal practice. It initially started by committing to expressing gratitude before getting out of bed, and a forty-day morning vinyasa flow practice and meditation. The vinyasa practice included an intense focus on grounding through the legs and tapping into my abdominal strength. I worked on these areas of the body because I felt shaken and pulled at my center, and my level of confidence was completely shot. I found a way to move that encouraged more creative transitions from posture to posture and the engagement of breath outside of the hatha practice, but more in line with my kundalini yoga roots. Through deep core and physically exhausting movements, I pushed beyond what I thought was possible for my body. I devoted two hours to the full practice, and after I came out of final relaxation, I did Alternate Nostril Breathing, sat in stillness for fifteen to twenty minutes, and then journaled. The moments of journaling typically connected to love and anything that popped into my head during meditation. Sometimes I could barely get through the meditation, and I returned to my twenties when I cried constantly. The practice was all about working through my pain and reconnecting to me. Within the practice I found trust, commitment, devotion, and love.

During this process, my teaching practices became a creative mash-up of my personal life. My sacred Spiritually Fly practice was a reflection of my family, church, Dr. Horton, kundalini *kriyas* (series of postures, breath, and sound), meditation, music, love, and the joyous flow of vinyasa. Outside of my morning practice, I also spent a lot of time writing. Words poured from my soul, and messages came in the form of quotes, poems, intentions, hopes, and dreams. It's true:

out of darkness comes light, and my light was a spiritual expression that looked very different from my childhood relationship with God.

WHAT ARE THE SPIRITUALLY FLY SUTRAS?

The word *sutra* is defined as "a collection or sacred thread of aphorisms." Individually they are powerful and dynamic, but threaded together they have the ability to inspire and ignite a personal revolution. Back in my modern-day cave, I identified seven principles that addressed my inner struggles, fears, and doubts, and each principle gave (and continues to give) me the strength to maneuver through life with more grace and harmony. The sutras help me stay true to myself, while simultaneously uncovering the delicate nature of my human existence. As I dance through the forever-changing landscape of life, I utilize these sutras as a way to stay dialed in to my soul and plugged in to the unique qualities of who I am.

My goal wasn't to create my own spiritual practice but to reconnect to a forgotten part of my being. I realized that when I fell in love and became involved in a chaotic relationship, I left a part of me behind. I left behind the part of Faith that questioned spirituality and was unafraid to explore God through dedicated practice. I ignored the intuitive side of Faith who trusted her gut and was willing to take a chance. Mostly, I dumped the loving qualities of Faith and placed them in the hands of another person. I knew this practice was what I needed to peel back the jaded layers and drop some habitual patterns.

From birth, our every action, experience, and intent are imprinted on our minds and hearts. As humans, we consciously and subconsciously absorb impressions—healthy and unhealthy. Over time, these impressions manifest into our individual tendencies or habitual patterns. Moments in time consciously or subconsciously dictate our actions, merge into our relationships, and rest deep within our essence. For example, I carried the healthy impression of having a supportive family, while at the same time, I also held the unhealthy impression of shame around my brothers' HIV-positive diagnosis. In Vedic philosophy, this concept is called *samskara*. As I committed to personal healing, I worked on releasing unhealthy samskaras and filling my mind and body with healthy impressions. Throughout the book, I will share a variety of methods, techniques, and approaches to purifying the mind, recharging the soul, and letting go of unhealthy impressions and making room for new healthy ones. As you move through, I will encourage you to explore your current impressions and invite you to create new samskaras through SoulPrints, which are daily action steps and personal commitments that support your path to personal elevation.

Within these pages, I will take you on a spiritual expedition of intimate stories, divine inspiration, and personal practices to healing. It warms my heart to offer my blended method of sorting through the struggles, realigning, and tweaking the spirit. In those moments when life is running smoothly and then the difficult and unexpected happens, I don't want you to fall to your knees and beg God for mercy. Instead, I want you to feel all the feels, acknowledge your current reality, and utilize the Spiritually Fly sutras and practices as a source of sacred strength and growth. My hope is that this book is the beginning of your journey to spiritual expansion. I also encourage you to use it as a point of reference and a guide to moving through your mysterious, sometimes messy, wondrous life.

SOULPRINTS: HOW TO USE THE BOOK

The soul is described by many religions and cultures as the embodiment of a spirit that is believed to give us life and that lives forever. It is the spiritual force within that provides us with our internal moral values, our emotional nature, and our deep-rooted ability to feel kindness. The soul is our divine self. Each chapter of this book taps into the magnificence of the soul and uses one of the sutras to amplify it. As you create new SoulPrints, you will cultivate your own sacred steps to designing a Spiritually Fly life.

The approaches I share in this book and continue to incorporate in my own life are specifically pulled together to help you cleanse, align, and fly. The idea is that as you move through your day, every act should be a reflection of your soul. If you are hurting, emotionally charged, and negatively compromised by unhealthy samskaras, it is impossible for you make personal choices that are true to your soul. In that state, you are unable to maintain healthy relationships, live mindfully, speak honestly, or simply feel a sense of joy. Although we all live in a cycle of detrimental imprints, we all have the capacity to shift and change.

Before you dive in, I feel it's important to share a few terms and concepts. This will make it easy to move through the sutras, process your personal work, and focus more on nurturing yourself. Described on the following pages are a few concepts and things to consider.

The Spiritually Fly Three Ms

As one of my teachers was going through my wellness training academy, a light-bulb went off in his head. He realized that what made a delicious Spiritually Fly class were what he called the Spiritually Fly three Ms: mantra, mudra, and meditation. When he began to merge the three Ms in his classes using my teaching approach, the students started to have a more spacious experience in class and off the mat.

Mantras are dynamic and mystical words formulated to transfer energy across space and time. The Sanskrit *man* means "the mind," and *tra* means "to transport." As a mantra moves through the mind and lips, you are able receive the power of the sound current. Within this book I use mantras from various teaching lineages to invoke the power of healing.

Mudra means "gesture" or "attitude." The entire body can be a mudra and generate a mood or expression that alters our consciousness. In each chapter, I will highlight a *hasta* (hand) mudra. When mudras are performed with the hands, the energy flows through the body and penetrates the mind. The hasta mudras will be merged with specific yoga postures or suggested with a meditation practice. I've found that mudras can be a beautiful source of inspiration and can easily heighten the power behind intentions.

Meditation is part of the global lexicon and is practiced anywhere and everywhere. Within these pages, I share meditation techniques that include visualization and breath awareness and some that merge mantras and mudras. Like all meditation practices, the key is not to get distracted by the distractions. Know that thoughts will float, and your directive is to let them float out with the breath or the next mantra.

Engaging the Body

Yoga practices in the form *asanas*, or yoga postures/poses, are shared at the end of each chapter and include both hatha and kundalini styles. The word *hatha* is broken into two balanced parts: *ha* meaning "sun," and *tha* meaning "moon." Energetically, a hatha yoga practice should feel balanced, and the mind and body should be in harmony. The majority of yoga styles taught within Western culture are hatha. These include Iyengar, vinyasa, Ashtanga, yin, restorative, and yes, power yoga.

Kundalini yoga, as many will say, is very different. First, the word *kundalini* refers to the energy that rests dormant at the base of the spine. When activated, through a variety of ways, it travels up the spine along energy channels associated with your mind, physical body, and soul. Kundalini yoga merges mantras or devotional chanting, meditation, physical movement, and breathing techniques to elevate your energy and strengthen your aura.

You will have the choice to follow one or both of the practices to see what resonates with you on a particular day. Each practice can be completed in an hour. My recommendation is to do the hatha practice first, then flow into the kundalini practice, unless I suggest otherwise within a specific chapter. You will also see the word *kriya* attached to a meditation or set of movements. *Kriya* has multiple meanings depending on the yogic style. Broadly speaking, it is evolutionary action. *Kri* means "action or effort," and *ya* means "soul." Within this structure, kriyas are practices designed to elicit a specific outcome that merges breathing techniques, poses, and sometimes mudras.

Journaling and Sacred Space

You will be offered prompts to journal throughout your Spiritually Fly journey. Journaling is a way to record where you've been but also how you are elevating. I recommend purchasing a journal specifically for your Spiritually Fly practices. In addition, if you can, create a mindful sacred space in your home or identify a sacred space in nature where you can read, practice, breathe, meditate, and journal. Wherever you choose to practice should feel safe and comfortable. Don't feel like you have to go all out; keep it simple and authentic to you. A yoga mat, pillow (any kind), and a thin blanket or basic bathroom towel will work fine. Or feel free to get fancy by adding a candle, incense, and essential oils to the mix.

Chakras: Wheels of Spiritual Healing

Throughout the book I will discuss and reference the chakra system. The work I do as an instructor and the approach I take with my own spiritual growth are based on the energies of the chakras. Often described as wheels or disks, chakras are dynamic energy centers aligned along the spine of all humans that directly connect to everything we are and desire to be. Originally discussed in the sacred temples of Egypt, it was believed that the flowing waters of the Nile River represented the backbone of the human body, and the temples were intentionally placed along the river to align with the chakras. In addition, many of the Egyptian deities are connected to these wheels of healing. The chakras also appeared in the teachings of yogic texts called the Vedas. The beautiful aspect is that within each culture, the chakras are the same, physically, emotionally, and spiritually.

This brief summary of the system provides the following for each of the seven main chakras: its name in Sanskrit and English; the position it occupies in the body; the Egyptian deity, sound, color, element, and qualities associated with it; and an affirmation.

1. Muladhara (Root): Located at the base of the spine around the first three vertebrae, this chakra is rooted by the strength of Osiris. Filled with the grounded, foundational earthiness of life, its sound is *Lam*, and its color is red.
   AFFIRMATION   *I am rooted, safe, and supported.*

2. Svadhisthana (Sacral): Flowing magically below the navel and above the pubic bone, the sacral chakra twirls the sensual creative channels with the sound of *Vam* and vibrates the color orange. Infused with the element of water and honoring the god Anubis (opener of the way), this realm holds our deepest emotions.
   AFFIRMATION   *I move with fluidity and grace.*

3. Manipura (Solar Plexus): Powered by the purification qualities of the goddess Sekhmet, the third chakra is located at the bottom of the rib cage and above the navel and is the place of self-confidence and self-esteem. Blazing the sound of *Ram*, its color is yellow, and its element is fire.
   AFFIRMATION   *I am a powerful being.*

4. Anahata (Heart): Saturated in compassion, forgiveness, and love, the heart chakra divinely ripples the sound of *Yam*, holds the color green, and governs air. I call this the middle sanctum because it is located at the center of the chest, which sits between the lower and higher chakras. Appropriately, the sky goddess Hathor reigns over the heart.
   AFFIRMATION   *I am open to giving and receiving love.*

5. Vishuddha (Throat): The lines of communication float along the blue shades of turquoise with the sound of *Ham*. Located at the throat, this chakra represents our ability to share thoughts and feelings with truth and grace, while also being an open and active listener. Composed of the qualities of king Djehuti, scribe of the gods, this center connects us to our inner truth and helps us cultivate ways to share it with the world.
   AFFIRMATION   *I communicate with ease and truth.*

6. Ajna (Third Eye): Sometimes called the "first eye between our two eyes," this magical point of indigo is governed by the glorious mother goddess, Isis. Radiating the sound of *Aum*, this is where wisdom, intuition, perception, and visualization sit.
   AFFIRMATION   *I listen to my inner wisdom.*

7. Sahasrara (Crown): Shining brilliantly from the crown of the head, this chakra glitters cosmic energy and the color violet. Blessed by the most noble Egyptian god Horus, this "gate of salvation" connects us to consciousness, and a pure awareness, and reveals our relationship with the divine source internally and externally. With a blissful nature of enlightened spiritual connection, this path opens us to the beauty of silence.
   AFFIRMATION   *I honor my divine light.*

Additionally, *nadis*, or streams of energy, run through and around the chakras. Within Tantric philosophy, the three most important nadis are the *ida*, the *pingala*, and the *sushumna*. The ida is the left stream representing the feminine/moon/omega energy that starts at the root chakra and winds its way up the spine to the left nostril. Like the ida, the pingala also twirls up the spine but represents the masculine/sun energy and ends at the right nostril. I refer to the sushumna as the "main line." It is the center stream in which kundalini energy moves up and through the middle of the body, root to crown.

Time and Commitment

As I shared, this is a journey of the soul, and in order for change to happen we must commit to the process. You will find moments where I encourage you to practice a specific meditation, yoga sequence, and journaling session for an extended period of time. I don't want you to feel overwhelmed, so I encourage you to start slowly. Commit to seven days at first, then fourteen days, twenty-one days, and so on until you work your way up to a forty-day commitment. The work of self-renewal is not immediate, and sometimes we have to press "rewind" in order to settle into the space of long-lasting transformation.

I truly hope you will incorporate these tools and techniques into your life and commit to breathing through the uncomfortable. As we move along this path together, keep in mind your life is not defined by past experiences or unhealthy choices. You have the capacity to reflect on your current state, create new impressions, and design a life that works for you. Enjoy moving through the book with an open heart and give yourself permission to dwell in the essence of your own spiritual connection. While some of the teachings may be ancient, and the approaches may be modern, they are all infused with a divinity that is uniquely Spiritually Fly!

Love is my only option,

a moment of softness
    poured over me
my heart felt gentleness
I finally let go

lead with love

While cloud-gazing in Malcom X Park on a Sunday morning, the poem on the opposite page came to me out of nowhere. The softness of the cloud formations blended effortlessly with the gentleness of the spring breeze in Washington, DC. It delivered a sweet moment where love rushed in and I surrendered. It somehow created cracks in a block of energy that stimulated a shift within my heart. Love didn't surface in the most blissful of circumstances, but instead, it twirled its way around one of the most challenging experiences in my life that was laced with abuse. Challenges creep in when you least expect them, and these unexpected flashes in time can deliver some the greatest insights in your life. Even when you think you are going to crumble, the light brightens your day, and you realize it's going to be okay. As thoughts drift in, you realize you are important, and the only way to feel better is to devote time to yourself.

Months before, I was caught in an emotional storm of a really bad romantic relationship, while at the same time attempting to live a life filled with hope. The person I was engaged to marry, whom I had loved for years, was no longer the light of my life, the man who made me laugh, or the "gentle giant" who supported me unconditionally. Over the course of seven years, our relationship gradually turned into a toxic, manipulative, and emotionally draining connection I could not maintain. It took me a year to leave him, and another two years of being alone to regain my self-worth. But on this particular morning under cumulus clouds, I began to feel the first step back to self-love and a rewiring of my heart. I began to process the meaning of love and contemplate life tempered with cool droplets of tenderness. With each inhale of a fluffy cloud, I exhaled "love yourself" into the earth. This simple ritual of the breath grounded me, and slowly reminded me of what's valuable. It reminded me that I had the capacity and the tools to return to my heart.

TALK YOUR HEART INTO BELIEVING

Two months before this personal realization, I found myself sitting on the steps of my apartment at 16th and Euclid crying frantically and dialing a local women's crisis center. My mind wanted to call my mother, but I knew she wasn't the right elixir for my soul. A lovely woman answered the phone. She immediately asked if I was physically safe, and if she needed to contact the police. My physical body was fine, but my emotional body was blazing with anger and fear. For over thirty minutes, we chatted, I cried more, and at some point we even laughed. The river of emotions flooding my heart gave me a moment of divine clarity. There was something special about talking to a complete stranger that enabled me to regain focus. The conversation allowed me to pause long enough to absorb the simplicity of my breath. All of her questions and each of my responses led to the truth. It was time for the relationship with my fiancé to end, and I desperately needed this connection to clear the smoky fog that surrounded my insecurities.

At some point you've probably gone through a bad love affair that resulted in heartbreak and massive disappointment. Or maybe you are in the middle of a messy love dynamic that you are afraid to end. It doesn't matter where you are. Toxic relationships are massively destructive, and they brutally destroy one's self-esteem. In your own relationships you may have thought the yelling, paranoia, unfair accusations, or random trips on the emotional rollercoaster were temporary. Then in the middle of fear, frustration, and rage, you asked yourself, "Do I deserve this?" Or you may have pondered, "How did I get here?" Even after those questions, you may have looked past the warning signs and talked yourself into believing things would change. The change in behavior isn't just about a toxic partner, it's also connected to your willingness to stay in the muck. Yes, your partner may have stripped away your self-esteem, but the red flags appear when there's a loss of self-worth and self-care. They intensify when you let go of the activities, interests, hobbies, and even quality relationships that make your soul shine.

Regardless of your relationship status, know you can only save yourself from emotional, physical, and spiritual annihilation by believing you are worthy of your own greatness. It's impossible to make sense of a poisonous relationship, and how it blindsided you. Trust me, it only creates more anxiety and emotional contamination. Instead, drop into you and cultivate a relationship with your heart. Take the time to pause, to find a place of inner softness, and to remember who you are. This is the start of your journey into the self.

CREATE A FOUNDATION TO BREATHE

Breathing is an essential component of life and is crucial to the practices of yoga and meditation. Without conscious breath flowing through you, it is impossible to absorb and feel the connection between body and mind. When you visualize breath moving into one area, your molecular structure will immediately shift, and as a result, your body responds positively. For me, the breath is my foundation for living authentically. It is the key that opens the door and gives me space to pause, reset, and fortify my connection to myself and others. I constantly share with my students the importance of having a daily breathing practice as a form of self-care. It is the same self-care we take in preparing a healthy meal or brushing our teeth. When breathing is approached with attention and devotion,

breath body soul
shedding the layers
unraveling the discomfort
letting go of yesterday
awakening to you

it becomes a habit that gives you time to pause. When you pause, you create pockets of time to reflect. When you reflect, you access your state of being, and in that, gratitude and self-acceptance turn into self-love. Basically, self-care has the amazing ability to ripple into self-love. When you activate deep care for yourself without compromise, you intuitively see what's in front of you with a neutral mind and open heart.

On a scientific level, conscious breathing allows oxygen to move more efficiently through the body, promotes concentration, and boosts overall vitality. It puts the body in a place of healing and changes the response of the body's autonomic nervous system. As the breath flows, it fires messages to the brain to make adjustments in the parasympathetic system, which slows the heart rate and generates a feeling of calmness in the sympathetic system. In moments of fear, anger, and even depression, the breath has the power to draw the body and mind into a place of harmony. Helping the body's systems to work properly through a daily breathing practice builds a strong immune system. I like to think that while eating, sleeping, and physical movement compose the framework of healthy immune function, breathing is the delicate yet solid force of nature that brings about stability. Along with helping to fight the progression of autoimmune diseases, conscious breathing lowers cortisol levels and blood pressure. Modern life has taxed our physical body, and even the basic function of driving a car compresses the spine and makes it difficult to fully access the diaphragm. When you make time to breathe and activate the diaphragm, you remove toxins and set a foundation for life. Breath is life, and conscious breath delivers a limitless life.

The three breathing practices described below will steady and calm the nervous system. While they are often taught during yoga classes, these techniques also blend smoothly with meditation and deep contemplative exercises and can be done anytime, anywhere.

UJJAYI BREATH

Typically translated as "victorious" breath and often called deep yogic breathing, *ujjayi* has been taught in the hatha yoga tradition for thousands of years as a method to link breath and body. When this linking occurs, the breath builds heat in the body, while also calming the mind. The Hatha Yoga Pradipika states that "ujjayi should be performed in all conditions of life, even while walking and sitting." This breathing practice relieves tension, encourages the flow of energy in the physical body, improves concentration, detoxifies the mind and body, and increases energy and the level of oxygen in the bloodstream. Mostly, it enables us to breathe through challenges, physical and emotional.

HOW TO PRACTICE   Come into a comfortable seated position on the floor or in a chair. Straighten your spine so the breath can flow freely. • Slowly inhale and exhale through your mouth. On the exhalation, tone the back of your throat by slightly constricting the passage of air as if you were trying to fog up a window. • Once this feels comfortable, apply the same toning of your throat to the inhales. Do this for a few rounds. • Now seal your lips and continue this same technique but this time breathe in and out of your nose. I often recommend breathing in and out on a 1:1 ratio, i.e., breathe out for the same amount of time that you breathe in. Keep the flow of your breath steady and smooth. • Do this for one minute. Return to a natural breathing pattern and notice how you feel.

ALTERNATE NOSTRIL BREATHING (*NADI SHODHANA*)

Nadi Shodhana, or Alternate Nostril Breathing, is another hatha yoga breathing practice that purifies the energy channel in the subtle body by alternating the breath between the nostrils. I like to call this breathing technique "the sweet spot" because it calms the mind and cultivates a balanced platform for the emotional body, while also effortlessly syncing with the physical body. As the breath moves from the left nostril (moon channel or feminine energy) to the right (sun channel or masculine), it improves mental performance, activates the parasympathetic nervous system, increases respiratory strength, and reduces blood pressure. Keep in mind, feminine and masculine energy flows through us all. When you think feminine, imagine self-reflection, introspection, and intuition. On the flip side, masculine can be considered logical thinking, digestion, and heat. The true quality of sweetness is that Alternate Nostril Breathing moves *prana* (life force energy) through the central channel of the subtle body bringing about an overall sense of equanimity.

HOW TO PRACTICE Sit comfortably. Place your left hand lightly on your left thigh. • Using your right hand, fold your middle and index fingers into your palm. Leave your thumb, ring, and pinky fingers extending out and up. This hand position is called Vishnu mudra and is named in honor of the Hindu deity Lord Vishnu who energetically represents preservation. • Use the right thumb to close off your right nostril and slowly inhale through the left nostril. Then close off the left nostril with your ring finger as your release your thumb and exhale through the right nostril. • Now inhale through the right nostril, then close it off with your thumb and exhale through the left nostril. This is one round of Nadi Shodhana. • Once you have it down, close your eyes and continue the technique for ten to twenty rounds. If this hand position is uncomfortable, place the middle and index fingers of your right hand on your third eye (between the eyebrows). • At the end, drop the right hand, and return to your natural breathing pattern through both nostrils. • Sit still for a few more minutes and observe your body and mind.

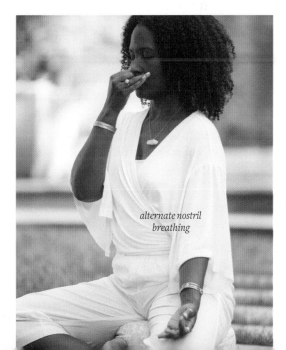

alternate nostril breathing

LEFT NOSTRIL BREATHING

Left Nostril Breathing is perfect for when you are feeling overly anxious, nervous, angry, or frustrated. When you breathe through the left nostril, a cooling, cleansing effect washes over the mind and in a matter of sixty seconds, you become calm.

HOW TO PRACTICE   Sit comfortably with a straight spine. • Place your left hand on your left thigh. Close off your right nostril with your right thumb, and keep your other fingers straight. Begin breathing slowly through your left nostril (inhale and exhale) with your eyes closed. • Keep your right nostril sealed throughout. Do this for one minute. • At the end, drop your right hand, breathe through both nostrils, and notice how you feel.

WITHIN THE LANGUAGE OF LISTENING, FIND STRENGTH

Humans are dynamic sound boxes bursting with primal resonances, words, and phrases and mental vibrations that ripple through our veins. Language is the way we think and the way we communicate. Like all sounds within the universe, the waves in our bodies travel along high and low frequencies, and they have the capacity to shift the way we think, feel, and respond. Verbal and visual, positive and negative, daily messages melt and merge into our subconscious mind. As our mind absorbs the messages, our brain catalogs the words and shapes the way we live and love ourselves. Self-loathing and self-destructive messages pierce the core of confidence. We start believing they are true, and past experiences blindly guide our present choices. We twist and grind our mind, hoping the inner dialogue will change or transform into something smooth. But this is not how transformation works; we have to put in the effort to reshape how we talk to ourselves, and coach our hearts through verbal recovery. When we activate healing technologies like sacred mantras and daily affirmations, we have the ability to release some of the negative thought patterns and create space for healing. This is the moment negativity starts to dissolve and *mukta* (liberation) pours in. Each day we awaken to limitless possibilities, but action must be taken for liberation and freedom to be experienced.

Self-loathing doesn't happen overnight. We all have something pressing against our hearts, whether it's some level of trauma or something we read on social media. The present experience often pulls us into the past where we felt inadequate, ashamed, or less than. Whatever the past circumstance, there's zero space in our short lives to spin the wheel of inner negativity. Take a second to think about how you treat and actively support your best friend. You shower your friend with compassion, praise their successes, and offer encouraging words when they are down. Mostly, you respect, honor, and love your best friend. Now think about what you tell yourself on a daily basis. Your inner messages may be disguised as lowering your bar, tough loving yourself, constantly highlighting your failures, or comparing yourself to others. This is typical behavior when self-care acts aren't cultivated, and self-love has vanished. The fortunate thing is that self-loathing and negative self-talk can shift, and we have the ability to change the station and vibrate a new sound.

There are defining moments where we make the choice not to repeat the past. We opt to dig in, lock down, and record a soulful sound of love and personal power. The ghosts of pain, hatred, and self-destruction haunt us daily, and there's always a random trigger or wave of emotional discomfort. The transformational work starts with positive acts that uplift your capacity to be your best self. The Queen of Funk, Chaka Khan, says it perfectly in the song, "I'm Every Woman." The sound current of the rhythm and her powerful words transcend race, gender, and economic status. I view them as a reminder of my power to be magnificent: "It's all in me." One night while dancing to this song as a way to pull myself out of negative self-talk associated with that toxic relationship, an inspirational pulsation flowed through me. I plopped on the sofa, and began to write Love Notes to myself. The first words that echoed through my soul were, "You are amazing!" Writing Love Notes is a technique that I share during workshops and women's retreats, but it isn't just another journaling exercise. Love Notes are meant to be seen and felt. They can be written on simple sticky notes or printed on your favorite paper. Once you write them, I recommend placing them in key locations such as your nightstand, mirror, desk, and refrigerator. Yup, the one on the refrigerator is very effective in maintaining a healthy diet and keeps you from emotional eating. If you have tons of them scattered around the house, I suggest pulling them together and creating one gigantic love note. Place it in a strategic location where you can see it multiple times a day.

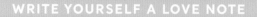

WRITE YOURSELF A LOVE NOTE

Set your timer for five to seven minutes, then sit comfortably or relax on your back. • Close your eyes and begin to breathe deeply. Allow your inhales and exhales to flow smoothly as you soften your body. Give yourself the time to pause and engage in an act of being just for you. • After ten to fifteen long deep breaths, begin to direct your thoughts around three words that describe what makes you amazing. • Try to stay open and connect to your compassionate heart and know these three words authentically reflect your awesomeness. Feel the energy around these three words. Visualize yourself engaged in life and submerged in the power of these words. Be a vessel for these words to flow through and around you. • When the timer goes off, open your eyes, take another deep breath, and immediately grab your pen and journal. Write down each word that came to you during the meditation and then use it in a positive sentence written in the present tense. For example, the word *creative* can be used as follows: "Creative thoughts flow through me with ease."

If this exercise was challenging, don't worry. I encourage you to repeat it daily for the next twenty-one days. You may notice that the words change, and of course, your state of mind will shift. I recommend doing this in the morning as a way to start your day grounded in self-love.

Love Notes are sugary reminders of who you are and desire to be. Over the years, my clients have described them as the tonic we all need to recharge the heart. So here's your opportunity to recharge yourself with drops of sugary self-love talk.

FORGIVENESS IS MY TEACHER, LOVE IS MY GURU

Forgiveness is one of the most divine expressions, based in and completely rooted in love. In order for us to give and lead from a place of love, we have to release hurt feelings and stop blaming ourselves when things go wrong. We all make mistakes, and there's nothing worse than holding on to the past and allowing it to negatively impact relationships (with yourself and others). After trauma, we naturally shield ourselves from future harm, and our fight-or-flight response kicks in when we're triggered. When the wall goes up, the emotional poison seeps deep into the subconscious, and this makes it challenging to fully love yourself.

looking back
feeling it
giving thanks
letting go
moving on

Forgiveness doesn't mean you will forget. It only means you have the power to release the anger, resentment, and frustration associated with a traumatic situation. There's an interesting intersection between stress, psychological health, and forgiveness. When you forgive, you naturally feel less stress when you recall a difficult situation, and overall your symptoms of depression and anxiety are greatly reduced. Forgiveness is the greatest gift you can give yourself. By acknowledging what happened and letting go of shame, you open a doorway to self-compassion and kindness.

The struggle we have with forgiveness is heavily saturated with the push-and-pull dynamics of disappointment. We hate ourselves for missteps and beat ourselves up even in moments of innocence. We are also plagued with the artificial safety of playing the victim or viewing ourselves as weak. Real talk: it's extremely challenging to forgive in the middle of pain, but when you've transitioned past the situation, free yourself and extend the hand of empathy. To shift, we have to fully commit to forgiving the person who caused harm and forgive ourselves. Once committed to the process, you can direct your focus on cleansing the energy surrounding the trauma, take responsibility for your part in the mess, and speak honestly to your spirit.

STEPS TO FORGIVENESS, JOURNEY TO LOVE

This exercise is one of the best ways to forgive and heal when someone you care for has caused harm. The goal is to provide clarity and move toward releasing the pain. Give yourself at least an hour. Find a location where you will not be disturbed and try to stay fully open to taking these first steps toward forgiveness. They may be difficult, but I have faith in you. Even in the uncomfortable moments, know you are making space for the good vibes to roll in. You are making space for love to saturate your essence.

HOW TO PRACTICE   Find a comfortable seat, place your palms face-down on your knees, close your eyes, and breathe slowly for about one minute. • Then using your right hand, begin to practice Nadi Shodhana, or Alternate Nostril Breathing (see page 19), for two minutes. • Then return your right hand to your knees, and sit in silence for five to ten minutes. • If thoughts begin to rush through your mind, it's okay. Simply bring yourself back to the present moment by breathing deeply in and out of the nose. Remain still and observe the breath. If silence is too much, play your favorite instrumental track. • Once you have completed the meditation, answer the questions below. This is a speed-journaling exercise, so grab a timer and take no more than three minutes to answer each question. Due to the sensitive nature of the questions and statements, pause and breathe before moving to the next. • At the end, feel free to go back and add more thoughts, but try your best to be clear and concise in the first three minutes. • Do this exercise weekly for at least three months. Select a day where you aren't rushed, and if needed, follow it up with a yoga class, brisk walk, or dancing. Moving the body after deep emotional work supports the effort and integrates it fully into the system.

- What does forgiveness mean and feel like to you?
- Who do you need to forgive and why?
- Why is it hard to forgive, and what are your triggers?
- How has the lack of forgiveness impacted your physical, emotional, and spiritual health?
- I forgive myself for . . .
- I forgive (name the person) for . . .
- I wish (name the person) well. Write a statement filled with kindness.
- Now that I am on the other side of forgiveness, letting go feels like . . .

WHAT IS LOVE?

Moving into a state of forgiveness takes constant effort and repetition. Negative thoughts and memories can easily distract us from moving forward. One of the biggest struggles is committing to a long-term plan of reestablishing love in the soul. The human mind is funny, but the beauty of being human gives us the capacity to be strong in our vulnerability. I often encourage clients to set emotional boundaries. If possible, during the forgiveness stage, disconnect from the person that caused harm. I also recommend that clients incorporate tangible elements into their lives that represent love such as the Love Notes and a daily breathing practice. But here's the major test of the heart: what is love?

In the late 1980s, American psychologist Dr. Robert Steinberg developed a triangular theory around love. His theory is based on three major components: intimacy, passion, and commitment. Intimacy is based on the feelings of closeness, connectedness, and bondedness. Passion includes feelings and desires that focus on physical attraction, romance, and sexual consummation. Commitment revolves around feelings that lead you to remain with someone and move toward shared goals. I'm sharing this because I want you to think about your love relationship with others, but mostly, I want you to contemplate your love relationship with yourself. Are there elements of intimacy, passion, and commitment present in how you show up for yourself? Are you deeply connected to your own soul? Are you passionate about who you are? Do you fully commit to personal goals? I honestly believe these three elements are essential to building a solid and loving relationship with yourself and others. I also believe there are many other components that dance along the lines of this triangle.

Life and practice guided me into reshaping my definition of and relationship to love, not just from the religious perspective of being Christlike, but from an inner spiritual place of true divinity. Divine love within my soul has given me the expanded capacity to forgive myself and others regardless of the situation or outcome. Blended with intimacy, passion, and commitment, my love paradigm is free, liberated, and joyful. But my refined definition of love is also devoid of expectations and judgment and more deeply filled with vulnerability and acceptance. Heaviness doesn't sit in the heart as long as there's passion and compassion for oneself. This requires us to clarify our needs internally and then commit to honoring our heart's truth by setting boundaries in all relationships, which enables us to drop into the breath of love with others.

So here's the approach. We constantly seek, desire, and place ourselves in situations to receive love. It starts in childhood. When we do something positive in the eyes of our parents, they typically respond with "I love you, and I'm so proud of you." More positive acts and accomplishments turn into more statements, expressions, and gifts intertwined with love. As we negotiate relationships in our teens and twenties, we start to layer on more intimate physical connections to love. In some cases, we start showing a physical expression of love in hopes of getting a partner or hearing those words come from their lips. This one-sided behavior destroys the internal framework of our innate spiritual ability to love unconditionally. It completely eats away at our soul because we are disappointed as a result of not getting what we want. It is human to desire love, but we should never compromise our personal beliefs and spiritual values for love.

As we all know, love bends our hearts in many directions; however, it is also a vibrating chemical eruption that occurs in the brain. It fascinates me how our cultural view of love completely contradicts our spiritual view. Culturally, we view and place love on a wildly romantic platinum pedestal of passion. We tell ourselves that if we give more love, then our loved one will change into the person we desire. Our jagged relationship with love also leads us to believe that love will overcome all the inadequacies in the other person. But really, it's not the other person who needs to change. Change is an inside job, and you are tasked with loving yourself with the greatest of effort, commitment, and devotion.

From my personal view unattached to organized religion, love is a choice rooted in compassion, understanding, and unconditional acts. Regardless of how you feel or how others act toward you, you have the ability to give and share love by choice. I'm not saying you can't get emotional about your position to give love or be in a state of love. I am saying that we should not allow our emotions to drive love, shape the way we give love, or modify the way we love and honor ourselves. I know this love approach is not sexy, but the act of giving and leading with love is fearless. It requires trust, which coats our hearts with the freedom to release the trappings of emotional lust. When we trust in our ability to love unattached to emotional desire, the burdens of forgiveness are easy to overcome. I share this perspective in the hope that you will live vibrantly from a place of love. I believe that stepping into forgiveness and trusting in your ability to reshape your relationships to the meaning of love will cancel out years of unhealthy impressions. Mostly, you will open the portal to loving yourself with intimacy, passion, and commitment.

THE LOVE SOUND BOX

Now I invite you to release your Valentine beliefs and follow me down a new road. This is an audible exercise to activate your vocal cords and take language off the paper and into your body to create cosmic waves of healing and empowerment. • Locate a place where you can speak these statements with a powerful voice. Remove your shoes, spread your toes wide, and stand firmly with your feet six to eight inches apart. • Take seven long, deep breaths. When you inhale, visually direct the positive energy through the body. As you exhale, imagine yourself surrounded by rays of golden light. • At the end of your seventh breath, say each statement five times out loud. Close your eyes while repeating the statements.

- I love myself unconditionally.
- I love who I am.
- Today, I choose myself.
- I am enough.
- I am love.

Do this as often as you need to to activate your voice and plug into your personal power. Along with hearing yourself, you are shifting the current and moving positive energy through the physical and emotional body. This practice pulls all of the elements of self-love together and automatically takes steps toward rewiring the mind.

yoga practice
giving love

Dedicate your yoga practice to giving and leading with love. Make a personal offering to yourself and those who are dear to your heart. Also send loving thoughts to a person you need to forgive. This heart-centered collection of postures and kundalini kriyas aids in balancing and harmonizing your energy rooted in compassion, forgiveness, acceptance, and lovingkindness.

mantra

Love is a divine
expression of my soul.

LOTUS MUDRA (*PADMA* MUDRA)   Before you start the practice, come into a cross-legged pose seated on a pillow or blanket. Bring your palms together at the center of your chest. Spread your fingers apart like flower petals and only allow the pinky fingers and thumbs to touch. Maintain this position for a few breaths and repeat the mantra to yourself at least three to seven times. Then be in stillness for another minute focusing on the meaning of the mantra.

Like a lotus flower that opens to the rays of the sun while its roots remain submerged in the mud, you have the capacity to rise from the muck of life and radiate beautifully. When activated with intention, the lotus mudra cultivates a loving attitude, eases loneliness, and releases tension.

CAT/COW (*MARJARYASANA/BITILASANA*)   Cat/Cow is a staple in most yoga classes. Typically done in the beginning as a warm-up for the spine, this posture has so many benefits that you may actually want to do it every day.

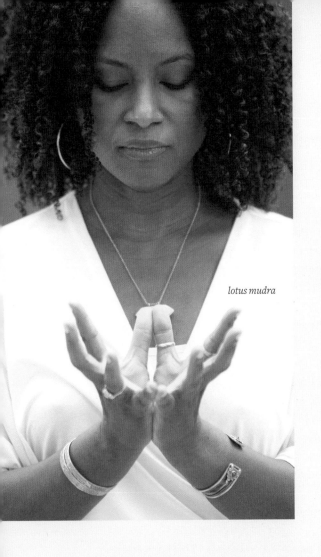

lotus mudra

The repetitive movements on the lower back and abdomen massage the muscles and internal organs. This process activates the adrenal glands at the top of the kidneys. The adrenals help with our fight-or-flight response, and the movements send a soothing signal to the nervous system. In classes I often guide my students through one to three minutes of Cat/Cow and say to them, "The arms are a beautiful extension of your heart." I do this because the motion releases tightness around the shoulders, strengthens the arms, and improves body posture by keeping the shoulders from rolling inward. As I mentioned, it stimulates the entire spine by aiding in the movement of prana, and this positive flow of energy moves into the neck where the muscles receive a stretch. For women, cat/cow reduces PMS symptoms, and, during pregnancy, conscious breathing while doing the posture calms the mind, which naturally supports the health of the baby. And just when you thought it couldn't get any better, this posture also improves blood circulation.

HOW TO PRACTICE   Come onto your hands and knees. Spread your fingers wide, wrists under your shoulders and knees under your hips. Your spine is in a neutral position with abs engaged. When you inhale, arch your back and lift your chest forward. At the same time the belly relaxes while the sitz bones spread apart. As you exhale, round the back in a catlike shape, drawing the belly toward the spine and the chin to your chest. Allow your inhale and exhale to initiate the movement and continue flowing in and out of the poses. Do this for one to three minutes. Be mindful not to swing your head vigorously.

SPHINX POSE (*SALAMBA BHUJANGASANA*)   A gentle and soothing backbend even for beginners, Sphinx Pose stretches the chest, shoulders, and lungs and lengthens the abdominal muscles. The gentle pressure on the belly stimulates the digestive organs and massages the kidneys. As you lift and hold the posture, you strengthen the spine and firm up the buttocks muscles. Firm glutes support the spine, hips, and pelvis. The Sphinx Pose provides invigorating benefits to the nervous system, and it's super therapeutic for those moments you feel mentally and physically fatigued. If you have lower-back issues caused by compression due to sitting or overworking the back, this pose can rebalance your natural curve and generate healing warmth.

HOW TO PRACTICE   Lie on your belly and place your palms and forearms on the floor with your elbows beneath the shoulders. Your legs extend behind you, and I recommend placing them about hip-bone distance apart. This position takes the pressure off the lower back. Press the tops of your feet into the floor and gently lift the kneecaps. Relax your shoulders and draw your shoulder blades back as you guide your heart forward. Your chin is parallel to the floor as you gaze forward. Breathe and hold the position for one to two minutes. Relax for five breaths by resting the entire body on the floor. Repeat two more times. While in the posture, continue to press your palms and forearms into the mat and engage your abdominal muscles.

Caution   If you are pregnant, definitely avoid doing this posture.

RECLINING BOUND ANGLE POSE (*SUPTA BADDHA KONASANA*)   This is my go-to self-love restorative posture. It immediately releases stress and encourages you to relax, which naturally impacts the parasympathetic nervous system. It is great for dealing with insomnia and creates a more meditative state of being by calming the mind. Because you are reclining and fully supported by the floor beneath you, and potentially props, it gently opens the chest, inner thighs, and groin. When we are afraid, angry, and frustrated, we automatically tighten in the hips, which restricts movement. It's okay to have a firm bum, but not at the expense of groin pain. This posture improves the flexibility of the groin and stretches the adductor muscles. Reclined bound angle is another delicious pose for pregnancy because of its relaxing effects. It also eases the symptoms of PMS. I always recommend drifting into this during the first few days of your moon cycle or in the moments when you feel hormonally out of balance and fatigued.

HOW TO PRACTICE   Lie on your back. Bring the soles of your feet together as your knees open to the side. Let gravity take over. The closer you bring your heels to the body, the more intense the posture will feel. If you feel too much pulling on your knees and groin, place pillows or blocks under your thighs. Rest your arms alongside your hips with your palms facing up. You can also place a pillow under your spine to elevate your chest and create more openness in your heart center. As an added touch, place a blanket over your body to provide a cozy feeling of self-love.

Caution   If you are pregnant, definitely use a blanket or pillow under your spine, while your hips remain on the ground. You should create a gradual incline. This position is not ideal for all stages of pregnancy, so avoid it if you are past thirty-four weeks, have a breech baby or hernia, or your pubic symphysis has shifted.

KUNDALINI KRIYA: CREATING SELF-LOVE

I love this practice because it fully taps into the magic of self-love. Through the hand and arm positions, it plugs into the heart center on a physical and emotional level, and it matches perfectly with the yoga postures in the previous section. It resets this realm of body and creates space for the good love to rush in. This kriya also directs energy to the crown of the head, which is associated with the pituitary gland. The pituitary gland is called the "master gland" because the hormones it produces control various areas of the body. When it is not healthy, it causes headaches, insomnia, changes in mood, depression, fatigue, reproductive issues (female and male), and unexplained weight gain. So for example, if you are unhappy with who you are, your brain sends stress signals to the rest of your body over and over. It becomes a steady infusion of personal toxicity. This kriya tackles that issue and provides a self-blessing effect while also correcting the magnetic field around the body. In addition, it activates everything from the navel to the throat and strengthens the heart center. I suggest adding this to your morning routine and doing it for at least forty days.

HOW TO PRACTICE   Open with the mantra *Ong Namo Guru Dev Namo* and then proceed through the following two phases:

PHASE 1   Sit in a comfortable cross-legged position and with a straight spine. Lift your right hand over your head with your arm bent and your palm facing down and hovering six to nine inches over the crown of your head. Your left arm

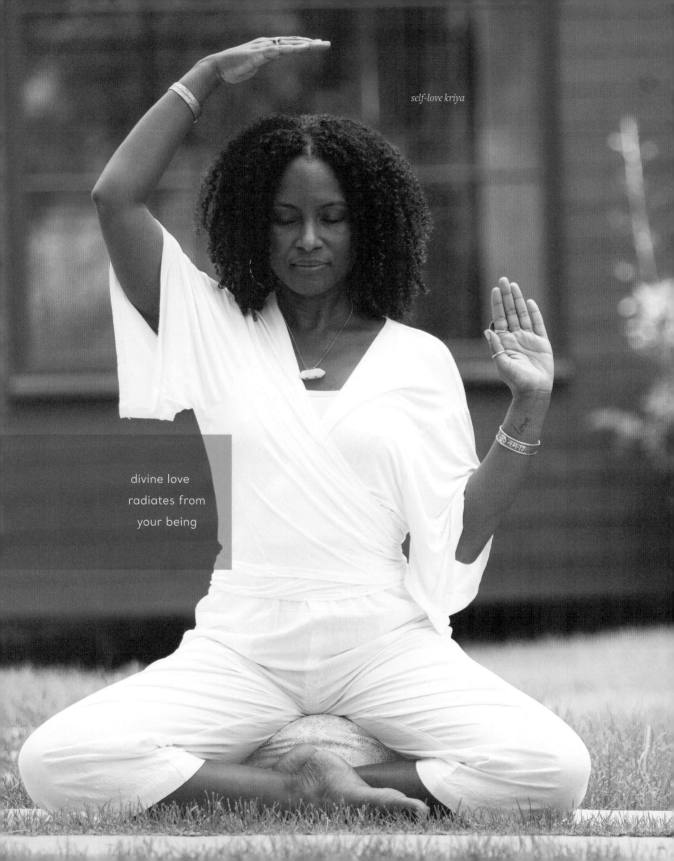

self-love kriya

divine love
radiates from
your being

is bent and held close to your rib cage with the palm facing forward as a gesture of blessing the world. Close your eyes, and focus your internal gaze on the lunar center, which is the middle of the chin. Take long, deep breaths, generating a sense of self-affection. Try your best to inhale for twenty seconds, hold for twenty seconds, and exhale for twenty seconds. Breathe and remain in this meditative position for three minutes. (In time, gradually work up to eleven minutes). Then slowly transition to the phase 2 of the kriya.

PHASE 2   Extend your arms in front of your chest, parallel to the floor, with your palms facing downward. Keep your arms straight as you continue to focus your internal gaze on the lunar center of your chin. Breathe slowly in and out of the nose. Take these long deep breaths for three minutes.

Then lift your arms straight overhead, fingers pointing upward, palms facing forward. Take long, slow breaths for another three minutes while continuing to gaze internally at the lunar center. At the end of three minutes, inhale and hold your breath for ten seconds with your arms still overhead and palms facing forward. Stretch the arms as much as you can and tighten all of the muscles in your body. Do this three times. Then rest your arms on your thighs and be in stillness for about one minute. Just sit still and observe.

Close this kriya with an extended *Sat Nam* mantra.

Your heart is a delicate lotus flower sitting in the muck of life, waiting for the sunrise. Dipping in and out of negative life experiences and wading through the murkiness simply pulls the soul deeper into the static behavior of self-destruction. The sun can be an inspiring choice to shift your thoughts and make a difference in your own life. Sometimes a traumatic situation kicks you into action, requiring you to make a choice to recalibrate. Once you feel the force, you can make a loving decision to breathe fully into you. When conscious breath creeps in, you make space on an intimate level, and you recognize the need to pause. In those moments, between the inhale and exhale, stillness grounds you, and you take steps toward shedding years of fear, anger, frustration, and mild depression.

The first few breathing practices in this chapter can magically peel back the heaviest of layers and pull you out of the darkest of holes. They make up the foundation for balancing the nervous system, calming the mind, and nurturing the body. Overall, conscious breathing is essential to everything you do and how you do it. It tells the mind not to react in difficult situations and gives you the tools to respond with grace and clarity.

Once breath control is learned, you easily gain the capacity to listen and reshape your inner voice. The audible inner voice is far more powerful than you can imagine. It cuts through the sound waves of outside voices and keeps you from being swayed by messages that contradict your intuition. There's a perfect pitch that resonates when you finally acknowledge your own worth. Positive self-talk creates a feeling that you are a good person, and you unapologetically treat yourself with respect. It surely takes a great deal of effort to clean the trash from your thoughts, but when you commit to loving yourself, you internally start to shift your own thought patterns.

Listening to the tenderness of your soul opens a doorway that leads to trust, compassion, kindness, and forgiveness. The depth of forgiveness frees the soul, grants personal liberation, and blossoms into self-love. Self-loathing washes away with each exhale, and light starts to shine. The light becomes nectar for the soul. This awakening turns into your highest connection to the self, which is the sweetest relationship you will ever have. Even in the midst of the uncomfortable, you have the strength to reclaim your voice, reshape your definition of love, and create a new soundtrack for your soul. These sacred vibrations make way for more personal intimacy, passion, and deep commitment. Purposeful intention and action allow you to feel your worth and root the process of retooling your heart in the truest form of love.

So regardless of where you are in the practice of giving and leading with love, know that it starts with the self. You were not put on this earth to endure pain and suffering, nor sacrifice all that you are for the sake of gaining love from outside forces. Your birthright is to experience the bliss and brilliance of life, bathe in the expansiveness of this earthly existence, and explore the nuances of what makes you human. And what makes you human is the ability to recognize love and navigate its waters with fluidity, and when the sky turns dark, you can safely return home to your heart.

my heart is heavy

my soul is weak

only devils hear my cries

silence kills the fruit

blood pours like sap

mud floods the gates of joy

melting waves cascade into sand drifts

kindness is only a wish

that my brother delivered from birth

love is a dream I wished for us all

my heart is cloudy

so I return to the darkness

where my soul finds comfort

where my mind hides

where connection to you does not rest

stand in your truth

i *hear my parents talking. The sound of my mother's voice cracks. I press my ear closer and closer to the wall, but I can't fully make out the words. The deep calmness of my father's voice filters in, "Okay, it's going to be okay." A few hours go by, my parents emerge from the bedroom. They bring Mark, Michael, and I together, and tell us that we're taking a family trip to New Orleans. My mother shared that I needed to take a blood test to determine if I was a carrier of hemophilia. I didn't think anything was odd, considering our family history. My grandfather, brothers, and a few male cousins have hemophilia. In addition, my mother was a carrier, and we were all too familiar with the complications and hospital visits related to Factor VIII deficiency. I figured this trip would be normal, and I knew I would be a carrier.*

The smell of hospitals always turned my stomach. The strange mix of industrial cleaning supplies and medical waste compounded with the fear pushed my heart into my belly. This day felt rather disconnected. My brothers' nurse, Karen Wolfe, was unusually distracted. She briefly chatted with us, then quickly ushered us into separate stations to draw blood. All of the adults, including my parents, were definitely on edge. My mother's gaze was drawn inward, and I honestly think my father smoked a pack of cigarettes in a matter of two hours. Even at eleven years of age I knew something wasn't right, and I didn't like it.

In 1982, my parents and thousands of others received a letter from the Centers of Disease Control and Prevention. The letter to my parents stated my brothers Michael and Mark might have been infected with HIV as a result of Factor VIII products. Hemophilia is a genetic disorder, and it has threaded its way through our family bloodline for generations. During the 1980s and '90s, my grandfather was considered the oldest hemophiliac living in the United States. Our family history of hemophilia was never an issue; however, upon receiving this letter, an intense level of panic rushed into our lives.

The death sentence of the letter and blood test confirmations coated our family with fear based on the stigma and societal beliefs around the disease. If you know the history of HIV/AIDS in America, you are aware of how many families were driven from their homes and local communities. The methods of HIV transmission weren't clear during the early days, and many people thought you could easily get infected by drinking from the same glass, using the same eating utensils, or even from a sneeze or cough. My parents were living in a state of constant distress, heightened emotions, and intense levels of control. Although I was young, I could feel the angst, and I quickly learned my role in the family. My job was to keep quiet and stay out of trouble.

My brothers and I were told not to share their status, for it was strictly a family matter. I vaguely remember my mother talking to our pastor, school officials, and a few other family members. Other than that, no one knew. People in the community definitely suspected something but just didn't say it to our faces. Everyone knew my brothers were hemophiliacs, and by the late 1980s, the media reported that over 10,000 hemophiliacs in the US were infected. People knew, and we were just lying to ourselves.

DROPPING STORIES TO REVEAL TRUTH

Adolescence is a time of transition and change, physically and emotionally. Cognitive, social, and sexual development is laced with the desire to be seen, heard, and accepted. Looking back I realize that it was during my adolescence that I began to keep lots of secrets. I was afraid, ashamed, and I wanted out.

Requiring children of any age to keep secrets can greatly impact healthy development and cause them to react and behave in an assortment of ways. Coupled with parental anxiety, it's no wonder that I opted in my tween heart to do my best to avoid being a problem. I played the role of the "good daughter" and focused madly on finding moments of freedom anywhere I could.

When parents/guardians are stressed, worried, or even consumed and not addressing their own issues like depression and addiction, children are left to design their own lives with limited connection to the self. Double lives are crafted when you have to hide the inner you. Lack of emotional maturity is hidden behind happy faces or pulled to the other edge through depression and anger. In addition, adolescents begin to craft their own methods of navigating life by engaging in behaviors that are high risk and self-harming. These could include the typical acts of sex and using alcohol and drugs, along with aggression, lying, extreme moodiness, depression, and drastic changes in appearance. Keep in mind, some of these are often modeled by parents. In my case, I was happy on the outside, confused and tortured on the inside, moody as fuck, and majorly depressed, and I lied about my home life on a regular basis.

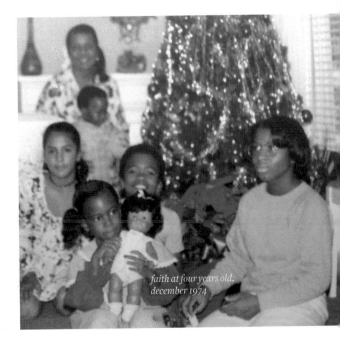

faith at four years old, december 1974

Being a teenager is damn hard, with or without social media, and internalizing our thoughts and feelings during these sensitive years can kick "crazy dust" all over adulthood. The desire to be popular and accepted by our peers transfers into adult behaviors such as addiction, releasing our power in relationships, and yes, more depression. I modeled my parents in relationships, and I never allowed intimate partners to know, see, or experience the real Faith. But the real modeling came in the form of not being honest with myself. As adults, we have the depth and emotional capacity to reflect and examine in our inner sanctum. We can choose to see ourselves clearly and unobstructed by the fancy, inaccurate stories we've built from childhood. As the stories are being built, we internalize them and cover reality with veils to hide divine, heart-centered truth.

One of the veils is the dishonest story of the victim. Without a doubt, if something traumatic happens as a child, we rely on our parents to come to our rescue and save the day. That includes being the best models they can be and setting us up to live vibrantly as adults. But if our caregivers have failed us in some way, we feel justified in the story we've shaped in our minds. This story can become the driver of our lives and paralyze our action to change, and in the hardest of times, we pull the story out just to feel comfortable, instead of feeling the tiny bits of pain clinging to the "real truth." Letting go of an old story and being honest with yourself is freedom. It's the sense of freedom I felt when I started to tell people about my brothers HIV status. The veil of shame and guilt slowly lifted, and the fear of disclosure softened each time I shared. On some level I became a model for my mother, inspiring her to be vulnerable and no longer a victim. The bizarre part is that it took her even longer to step into her truth: more than ten years after the death of my older brother.

Revisiting and acknowledging events in our past supports mental and emotional shifts. But mostly, it gives us a foundation from which to move forward and upward. The "Past, Present, and Future Journaling" exercise on the following page is ideal for quickly assessing how some of your childhood experiences impacted your adulthood. It's also an initial glance at where you've been, how you can cultivate stability in your truth, and how you can use this knowledge to cocreate your "Flyhood." Flyhood is when you are divinely living, fully in love with yourself, grounded in your truth, navigating the smooth and shaky with an open heart, and doing it all with a super-strong trust muscle.

BALANCING COMPASSION AND TRUTH

Telling the truth can be extremely uncomfortable and sometimes highly painful for you and others. Does that mean we avoid telling the truth in an effort to block the discomfort? Do we only tell half of what is true and leave the awful elements in the dark? All spiritual practices list truthfulness and honesty as primary ways of connecting and getting closer to God, or the Divine. I'm sure you've

PAST, PRESENT & FUTURE JOURNALING

Before beginning this exercise, take five to ten minutes to breathe and meditate. Promise me: don't read the questions below before you meditate. I want your thoughts to be fresh and free of stories, and I need you to be fully honest in your responses. As you answer the questions, clearly state your feelings and allow your vulnerability to flow. Go deep and know you are being held by the love within your own heart.

YOUR PAST: CHILDHOOD

- What episodes or experiences during childhood caused you to view those years as uncomfortable or miserable?
- What stories did you tell your childhood peers about your life that wasn't true?
- What were your coping mechanisms during this period?

YOUR PRESENT: ADULTHOOD

- What behavior(s) do you display when you are triggered by uncomfortable childhood memories?

- How do you cope with life when you are triggered by these memories?
- What is the story you continuously tell yourself to feed your fear, anxiety, or personal hatred so that you have to shift, move, or feel emotionally uncomfortable?
- Have you taken steps to find closure around the experience(s)? If so, did you find that closure?

YOUR FUTURE: FLYHOOD

Close your eyes for two to three minutes and think about how you could appropriate these triggers in a grounded and more balanced way.

- List ways you can respond gracefully rather than reacting negatively when you are triggered.
- What self-care techniques can you use when you are triggered?
- What is one activity you can do daily to celebrate your current life and reality?

experienced truthful conversations that felt like hell—the emotional distress lingered for days, and you were far from feeling spiritually awakened after the dialogue. Instead, you would have preferred not to have had the conversation or opted for dishonesty because at the time it felt easier.

Avoidance is simply pushing the truth into the ocean and walking away with the belief it will not return to shore. This and the telling of half-truths are delusional states of being that keep us trapped in fictional realities designed to numb the pain. Culturally we've been taught at every touchpoint of our lives that blaming others and avoiding the truth feels better. This is partially the result of not being equipped to responsibly deal with difficult situations and conversations in an honest and mature manner. From listening to our parents yell to breaking up with someone via text, we mostly avoid the truth as a way to protect ourselves.

As much as they enjoy the love and light aspects of Eastern philosophy and organized religion, many seekers gloss over the fact that they have to do the deep personal work in order to fly. Meaning the path is there, but they've chosen to jump forward and soar like a unicorn without a horn. Within the Yoga Sutras, there are eight limbs or branches of the "yoga tree." One of the limbs is composed of the *yamas*, which are ethical suggestions on how to behave and engage with the world around us. They include *ahimsa* (nonviolence—physical, mental, and emotional), *satya* (truthfulness), *asteya* (nonstealing), *brahmacharya* (continence), and *aparigraha* (nongreed or nonattachment). Like day and night, the teachings are intimately linked; one does not exist without the others. So in order to fly, we must breathe, feel, and experience all sides of our spirit in its human form.

For instance, ahimsa and satya cannot glide along the path without each other, so in order to talk truth, we must discuss nonviolence. In Sanskrit, the word *ahimsa* is derived from *a* meaning "not" and *himsa* meaning "to cause pain." Our goal is to avoid causing pain—physical, mental, or emotional—and instead cultivate kindness and a compassionate attitude toward ourselves and others. In the purest sense, *sat* means "that which is or exists." Satya essentially means to be honest in all you do. Although we may not know the full truth, we are definitely clear when we are sharing what we believe is the truth.

The tricky part is balancing these two teachings. Take for example an instance where telling your truth would cause harm to someone else. If you practice satya in such a situation, how can you practice ahimsa at the same time? Should you be honest even though you know it might be hurtful, or should you hold back and avoid causing pain? This concept can easily be experienced in the body during a yoga posture. When you are in the middle of a challenging pose, the mind will go through an internal dialogue that says hold, draw back, or push forward to a place of overdoing.

Off the mat, it can be really hard to practice this concept, especially in difficult circumstances such as the example above. When I first read the Yoga Sutras in college, I completely disregarded this concept, almost in the same way I disregarded it in the Bible. I said to myself, "It is impossible for me to be completely honest; no one on earth can do that." Over time I discovered that my approach to filtering and selective-information sharing was my reality in daily life. Basically my dishonesty traveled the path of personal motives and selfish desires.

THE TRUTH IS WHERE YOU ARE

Honesty is a fundamental principle to seeing yourself clearly. As a core value of all spiritual practices, honesty creates a deep level of trust with yourself and others. It creates a solid foundation for cultivating strength, and it holds you spiritually responsible for your actions. As a child I found it interesting that my mother would go to church almost every Sunday but continued to encourage us to keep the family secret. That meant that any time someone would mention or ask, we should say nothing. Ultimately, she was living and guiding us on a path that was on very shaky ground. Even today, where the levels of racism, sexism, and homophobia still float alongside modern freedoms, I fully understand where my mother was coming from. Yet, her real issue was never taking the time to be in a place of silence with herself.

Practicing yoga asanas has always supported my ability to engage in meditation. In those moments of silence, the truth is always revealed. That's the beautiful yet scary part about being with only your mind to keep you company. You can't hide or dodge who you are or what actions you took in the past. Your thoughts follow you like baby ducklings following their mother. Each one in perfect step with the other, enabling us to make our desired choices in life. As you know, and have probably felt by now, meditation is extremely effective in generating internal shifts. Having had an active meditation practice for the past twenty-plus years and teaching various forms, I've seen how sitting with oneself creates a different lane for living. When you commit to a forty-day meditation practice, especially some of the intentional kundalini meditations, a vast range of emotions travel to the surface. I've noticed how selfish statements and dishonest actions of the past have held me and others hostage, almost in the same way my parents were trapped in their own emotional struggle. Each day becomes a baby step toward standing and living in truth, regardless of how it feels.

In the silence
I hear
roars of truth.

But through all the sitting and contemplation of the truth, it all comes down to deciding what is or what isn't truth. Either you are truthful or you are not. There's no middle ground. Or is there? Even in those hard moments when you have to let go, the mental choice to speak from your heart is difficult. As a teacher, healer, and spiritual guide, it can be hard to sit and stand in a place of truth. Speaking the truth about my family comes easy now; however, stepping into my personal space of truth is still a challenge. For women or anyone that grew up with adults telling you to keep quiet, it can be grueling at times to be blunt and speak up.

Life is filled with unexpected moments, pain, loss, and heartbreak, but we have a choice to linger in misery or celebrate the good things.

You may often hear Buddhist teachings say that we create our own suffering. I definitely believe in this perspective. Holding on to our thoughts and feelings, even in meditation, can cause internal pain and struggle. This mental battle traps the mind and pulls at the soul. "Sitting on it" can increase your levels of worry and stress. It can also cause physical complications in the abdomen. This physical manifestation results in disease, frustration, and emotional disconnect. In this moment you are no longer aligned with your truth. So really, there's no middle ground. The truth is where you are, and you have no other choice but to walk the path of elevating your soul.

Many of the numerous students I've worked with over the years found it hard to tap into their own source of truth. Through journaling exercises they uncovered the blocks and their sources, but for some reason they couldn't share how they honestly felt with others. One of my clients remained married for years because she was unable to tell her husband that she was no longer in love with him. She feared social embarrassment, but mostly she didn't want to disappoint him or their children, extended family, or friends. Along with a daily asana practice, weekly therapy, and a 120-day meditation practice, she managed to find the strength to have an honest conversation with her husband and get a divorce.

Her 120-day meditation practice was focused on her throat chakra (Vishuddha), the energy center that honors personal expression and communication (listening and speaking). Since this chakra is related to the element of sound, I felt that having her do a meditation that involved chanting a mantra that incorporated the *bija* (seed) mantra for this chakra, *hum*, was exactly what she needed. In addition, I advised her to wear a blue gemstone such a lapis lazuli, sapphire, or topaz. Blue is the color associated with the throat, and it was crucial to plug in to as many sources as possible to use as tools for her shift. During our consultation, she also revealed that she was having thyroid issues. The throat chakra also supports a balanced thyroid, which impacts the central and peripheral nervous systems, heart rate, breathing, body temperature, weight, cholesterol level, and so much more.

The following meditation is a good way to activate your throat chakra and improve communication, especially when it comes to sharing the truth.

MEDITATION FOR THE THROAT CHAKRA

Sit in a comfortable position, with a straight spine. Rest the backs of your hands on your knees and form the *gyan* mudra by bringing your thumbs and index fingers together while keeping the other fingers straight. Energetically this mudra increases concentration; builds mental sharpness; stimulates the nervous system, wisdom, and receptivity; and aids in calming the mind. Focus your eyes on the tip of your nose and chant the mantra *Humee Hum Brahm Hum* for eleven minutes.

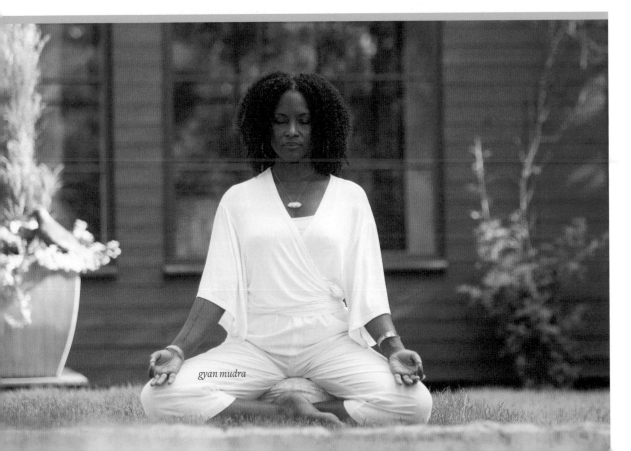

gyan mudra

SACRED MOVEMENT OPENS A PORTAL OF HONESTY

When I was a child, dancing was a significant part of my life, and the only place I felt safe and whole was in the twirls of motion. I vividly recall taking my tiny cassette player into our fancy living room and dancing for hours. Oddly enough, performing on stage also provided the same sensations. Feeling the vibrations of sound rip through my body opened portals to freedom and uninhibited thoughts and magnetic connections to God. Even in the midst of hating God, I felt a strong pull toward something that was more powerful than I could ever hope to be. The pulsating heartbeat and the creative blends of transitions, folding, opening, spinning, and falling were cosmic doorways. I only know this was my truth, and my inner alignment linked to the depths of my soul.

Truth starts from within! In order to stand and live in my truth, I've had to become completely honest about my abilities and levels of comfort and discomfort, and ultimately I've had to be clear about who I am at the core. It has taken years to step into this place, and even now, it is a daily practice. Having the inner capacity to wake up every morning and refuse to live in untruths can be challenging. In the vibrant face of social media, we unconsciously create an online image painted with a brush of what we desire or disdain.

Many years ago I only shared my unicorn dream of life. I almost never revealed the shadows of pain, shame, and insecurity. In the evolution of the Spiritually Fly sutras, I realized this was not who I was, and I was not standing and living in my truth. I'm not saying you have to share all of your life online, but it is essential to your emotional health to share honestly with yourself and others. I always encourage my yoga teacher trainees to share with integrity and from a place of personal values and offer content that inspires and uplifts, causes others to think about their own lives, and opens lines of communication in a world where technology has created disconnection.

Being in the flow of the physical body can be a beautiful mechanism to connect to truth and a great way to set the stage for your life. When you are vigorously moving, you consciously let down the walls and let God in. I know this is why I gravitated to the vinyasa yoga practice after meditating and practicing kundalini yoga for several years. Dance classes were no longer part of my daily routine, and the only form of vigorous movement was dancing at the club. Vinyasa yoga, like ballet and modern dance, provided a clear space for me to express, feel, and experience without being guided mentally in a particular direction. Creative and ecstatic movement merged with sound harnesses the energy within, releases negative vibrations, and generates a meditative flow of communion with spirit.

For the sake of understanding my connection to spirit, I want to share a little African history around dance/movement as worship. In every ancient culture, sacred dance has served as a ritualistic journey to connect and honor a higher energy. Our ability to transcend our human physical form is directly related to our emotional ability to "dance like no one is watching." I know that's probably not what our African ancestors were thinking, but sacred dance enables us to fully integrate the physical, emotional, and spiritual aspects of human existence. According to Kariamu Welsh-Asante in *African Dance: An Artistic, Historical, and Philosophical Inquiry*, there are three stages of African dance: invocational, transcendental, and celebration.

Invocational dance is the preliminary stage of calling on God. While it isn't the first form of acknowledging the Divine—it comes after the initial acts of invocation—but the dance heightens the devotees' connection and transports the spiritual process upward. I find it fascinating and uniquely in parallel with the vinyasa practice in that the invocational segment moves slowly and there's an element of body purification. In addition, this experience reminds me of the subtle bodies described in Vedantic philosophy, specifically the *Taittiriya Upanishad*. These subtle bodies are called *koshas*, or sheaths. We all have sheaths, and as we slowly peel them away, we get to the heart and depths of our soul. In the beginning of the yoga practice we are aware of the *annamaya* kosha, the outer sheath of the physical body (muscles, bones, skin, and organs), and the *pranamaya* kosha, the energy sheath related to breath. The mindful movement of breath and body give way to these sheaths and open a doorway to the next stage of diving deeper.

In the movement
I feel my truth.

As movement continues, transcendental dance, or "dance of the heavens," progressively shifts the energy, and the devotees become a medium of the Orixás. While the Orixás can be described as the demigods or deities of the Yoruba people, they are also found within various West African traditions, and African slaves carried these traditions with them. I'll share more details about the Orixás and the African diaspora in chapter 7.

On a personal level, I find that the Orixás are more than your typical mystical deities because they have the divine ability to arise within earthly beings and support the convergence of spiritual alignment. During the transcendental

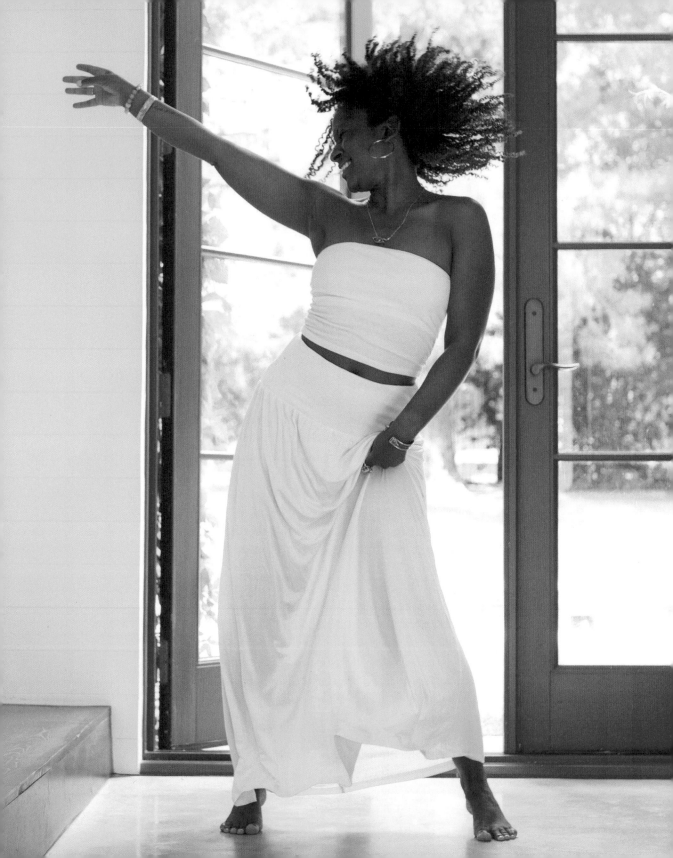

dance, an Orixá takes over the body and moves the dancer into an altered state of consciousness, which can bring about more powerful movement or subtle changes, but either way, an emotional release occurs that goes beyond space and time. Within the practice of yoga and meditation, the *manomaya* kosha (mental sheath) and the *vijnanamaya* kosha (wisdom sheath) begin to soften, and this clears a path to oneness.

The celebration dance seals the service and gives honor for devotion. As I drift into stages of the *anandamaya* kosha (bliss) during seated and closing postures and then finally rest softly in atman, my soul performs its own dance of celebration. There's an amazing physical release, a focused sense of mental clarity, and an element of internal healing in the soul. With clarity and healing comes an understanding of myself and a commitment to personal integrity. As always, the movements I practice and teach on the mat cultivate personal truth and strength, but the real work happens when you have to deal with unexpected obstacles that challenge your power to be and stand in your truth.

DANCE RITUAL

Now is the time to give yourself the freedom to dance it out and be in the flow of whatever comes up. Turn on your favorite playlist and dance uncontrollably for ten to fifteen minutes. I recommend using tracks that have indigenous drums in the mix. As you dance, feel your feet and legs rooting into the earth. Imagine the earth recharging your physical body and stimulating every inch of your soul. At the end of your dance session, pause and stand balanced on both feet. Close your eyes and feel the sensations moving up and down your body. As you stand there, give honor to Mother Earth for giving you the strength to stand in your truth.

yoga practice
moving with honesty & truth

Movement and stillness have always served as methods to peel back the veils we wear, the stories we tell, and the truths we hide. There's really no other way to flow in life than to be true to yourself and to stand authentically in your soul. Being in a place of truth doesn't come easy, nor does committing to living in your truth regardless of the outcome. The yoga asanas below and the kundalini Sat kriya that follows them will cradle and firmly hold you through the journaling and the forty-day meditation practice. Use this practice to move gracefully through your truth.

mantra

I live in truth.

MOUNTAIN POSE WITH LATERAL STRETCH (*TADASANA URDHVA HASTASANA*)   Taught and often glossed over in so many flow or vinyasa classes, Mountain Pose is active and energetically dynamic. I get so excited when I teach this foundational yoga posture because it gives me the opportunity to connect students to the power of a practice focused on personal strength, grounding, and inner stability. It improves balance and overall physical posture, increases personal awareness, and calms the mind. While giving space for the breath to flow through the body, it improves mobility in the feet, strengthens the legs and hips, firms the abdomen, and engages the buttocks. In addition, with the lines of energy moving up and down, it encourages healthy digestion, relieves tension throughout the body, improves blood circulation, and increases energy.

Adding a lateral stretch with the arms over the head elongates the sides of the body, shoulders, and armpits.

HOW TO PRACTICE   Stand with your feet slightly apart with the inner arches parallel to each other. Spread your toes apart and as they release into the floor, distribute the weight evenly between both feet and between the ball and heel of each foot. It helps to rock back and forth to feel and bring awareness to the distribution of weight. Engage your legs by lifting your knee caps and firming your thighs, and at the same time engage your core muscles and lengthen your spine by extending the crown of your head toward the heavens. As your abs engage, feel your tailbone naturally release toward the floor. Don't tuck your pelvis. Honor the natural curve of your spine. Keeping your chin parallel to the floor, slowly lift your arms overhead with the palms facing each other. If it feels comfortable, bring the palms together. Keeping your shoulders relaxed, lift your arms up a little more and slowly stretch to the left. Your chest remains forward and open. Hold the posture for five breaths as you experience a deep stretch through the right side of your body. Repeat three times on each side. While you are stretching and transitioning to the opposite side, keep your feet planted evenly on the floor.

LION'S BREATH (*SIMHA PRANAYAMA*)   There's a pose that goes with this breathing technique, but we are going to combine it with Cobra Pose instead (see below). Lion's Breath amplifies the throat chakra by harnessing the strength of a lion and inspiring us to roar. It releases toxins on the exhale, increases energy flow, and stretches the muscles of the throat, neck, and face. Lion's Breath also relieves tension and tightness, and in yoga class I also find that it breaks the seriousness of a moment and encourages students to let go.

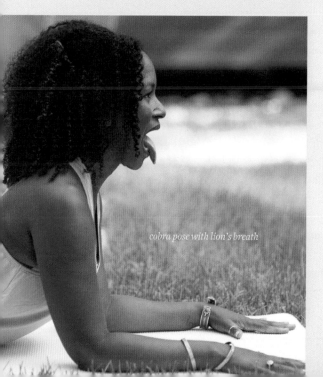
cobra pose with lion's breath

HOW TO PRACTICE   In a comfortable seated position, close your eyes and take three deep breaths through the nose. On the third breath, stick out your tongue, open your mouth really wide, and exhale forcefully from your mouth. Do this three to five times and create a loud lion's roar from your belly.

COBRA POSE (*BHUJANGHASANA*) WITH LION'S BREATH (*SIMHA PRANAYAMA*)   The perfect posture for increasing the flexibility of the spine, Cobra Pose also stretches the chest and enhances spinal and shoulder stability. Like most backbends, it energizes, which helps with fatigue, reduces stress, opens the lungs, and stimulates digestive and other abdominal organs. If you have carpal tunnel or are pregnant, I recommend keeping it safe by practicing Camel Pose (see next posture) instead.

HOW TO PRACTICE   Come to rest on your belly with your forehead touching the floor. Extend your legs behind you with the tops of your feet on the floor, and your legs hip-bone distance apart. Place your hands on the floor beneath your shoulders and spread your fingers apart. On the inhale, press into your palms and slowly lift your head and chest. Keep your elbows slightly bent and gently hug them into the body. Firmly press the tops of your feet and thighs into the floor and engage the abdominal muscles. When you feel more secure, lift up higher. Keep your thighs on the floor and the buttocks firm but not hard. Keep your shoulders relaxed, chest open, chin parallel to the floor, and gaze forward. Hold the pose for two slow breaths, release, then repeat two more times. Rest for one minute, then repeat three more times using lion's breath twice during each cycle.

CAMEL POSE (*USTRASANA*)   An expressive and heart-filled posture, Camel expands and stimulates the throat and heart chakras. Since these are two very sensitive realms of the body energetically, I believe this should be a staple in your yoga practice. With energizing effects, Camel addresses fatigue, improves respiration, stimulates the endocrine glands, and helps with digestion and constipation. It stretches the thighs, groin, abdomen, chest, and throat. For women, Camel releases tension in the ovaries and menstrual discomfort.

HOW TO PRACTICE   Come into a kneeling position with your knees hip-width apart and your thighs perpendicular to the floor. Direct your thighs slightly inward and firm up your buttocks just a little. For beginners, I recommend curling your toes under, but you can also release the tops of your feet down.

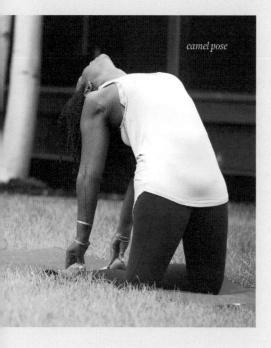

camel pose

Press your shins and tops of your feet firmly into the floor. Place the base of your palms, fingers pointing downward, on the tops of your buttocks. Use this position to spread your pelvis and guide the tailbone down. Inhale as you lift your chest. Exhale as you slowly lean back drawing your shoulder blades together. Beginners, keep your chin softened at the chest and your hands in place. To go further, release your hands to your heels while continuing to press your pelvis forward. This can be done one hand at a time or both at the same time. Just remember to move slowly and breathe. Your head can remain in position, or you can slowly extend it back to open your throat. Breathe here for five breaths, then carefully lift out on the inhale. If your head is back, rise with your heart first. Rest your hips on your heels for three to five breaths, then repeat two more times. At the end of the third round, return your hips to your heels and fold forward into Extended Child's Pose (see chapter 7). Rest here for ten breaths.

KUNDALINI KRIYA: SAT

Known as one of the most powerful, transformative, and complete kriyas within the kundalini yoga practice, the Sat kriya works on all levels of who we are—body, mind, and soul. By stimulating the natural flow of energy throughout, it balances the chakras, massages the internal organs, and strengthens the heart through the rhythmic pumping of the navel center.

HOW TO PRACTICE   Sit on your heels. If this is uncomfortable, place a blanket between your heels and your hips or sit on a pillow with your heels outside the pillow. If there is still too much pressure on your knees, sit with your legs crossed or in a chair. Extend your arms overhead and bring them close to the sides of your head. Interlace your fingers, extend your index fingers, and cross your thumbs—left thumb on top for a feminine energy, right thumb on top for masculine energy. Close your eyes and gaze at your third eye. Keep this position throughout the kriya.

Now chant the mantra *Sat Nam* at a steady rhythm, drawing the navel in and up toward the spine when you chant *Sat* and relaxing the belly when you chant *Nam*. Throughout, maintain a firm root lock. (Root lock, or *Mula Bandha*, is a diamond collection of muscles between the pubis and sitting bones. The lock can be engaged by contracting those muscles, lifting in and up.) Allow the breath to regulate itself. Do this for three minutes.

To end, inhale, hold the breath for five to twenty seconds, lift up while squeezing the muscles in the body, and focus on the crown of the head. Exhale completely and relax.

Standing in the truth takes love, bravery, and compassion, not just for yourself, but for the darkest moments of your life. When we look back on our experiences from childhood through a lens of examination, not blame, we can get clear on how those experiences poured into adulthood, and the many ways they dictated our choices and view of life. Even cloaked in the emotional veil of playing the victim, we have the capacity to unpack the shame and dig ourselves out of the guilt. In that phase of personal awareness, a stage is slowly being built for shifts into Flyhood. That's when you are entering a place where love, openness, and personal freedom can soar.

As we understand the broader dimensions of truth and how half-truths and avoidance move along the same path, we realize that there's a reason why truth is part of all spiritual teachings. It's a fundamental principle of knowing what is and how dishonoring the journey and not facing or telling the truth causes harm to oneself and others. Through meditation and contemplative practices, the truth always bubbles to the top. In the silence and stillness there's no middle ground; the truth is truth. But in understanding the heaviness of not speaking up, we must utilize all the tools available to strengthen the energy of communication. Working on the throat chakra is a must when it comes to truth and honesty. Along with addressing the physical and energetic misalignment of holding back the truth, throat chakra stimulation can readjust, purify, and blast through the blocks.

Using sound frequency and hearing your own voice is another path to living in your truth.

When things feel stuck, and you need to shake it out in order to sit and be still, I always recommend dancing like a crazy person. In Western culture we view it as a method or technique of simply moving the physical body, but in African and other indigenous cultures, it is a form of communicating with the Divine. Releasing the outer layers, letting go of old stories, and revealing the truth of our soul deepens our relationship to the self and gives us the strength to be honest with others. Ultimately, it gives rise to Flyhood! Finally, stepping into a place of honesty and standing in your truth isn't about forcing, demanding, or towering over others with THE TRUTH. It's about checking in with yourself, understanding who you are on a soul level, and living honestly in the world with personal conviction and intention.

Before we transition to the next chapter, I want to leave you with a few final tools. These are my Daily Acts of Honesty. They serve as simple methods of dealing with all that shows up when we feel the old stories of shame and guilt move into the conscious mind. These very basic acts will shift your perspective on how you deliver the truth and how you communicate your needs, wants, and desires from a place of honesty, and they will help you to feel more secure about your thoughts and words.

Daily Acts of Honesty

- Be thoughtful and mindful of the words you speak (verbal and written).

- Take your time when writing texts or emails, especially when you are upset or triggered. Pause, breathe, write, pause again, review, and send. If you are really heated, I recommend giving yourself at least an hour before sending.

- State your truths clearly, mindfully, and with intention.

- If your words could potentially cause harm to another, think about how you can maintain a high level of honesty fused with compassion. Tact is everything.

- When you are really upset or trapped in a situation, try your best not to react. It's okay to be angry, and you don't need to hide what you are feeling, but try to respond with purpose, clarity, honesty, and grace.

- Don't feel guilty after you speak your truth.

- Accept the consequences of hearing and sharing the truth. Trust me, it may hurt initially, but in the long run, you will feel better.

- Be honest with yourself!

breathe into your past
release the shame
as lessons prepare you for the next

breathe into your present
drop in deep
feel the stability elevate you

breathe into your future
ride waves of dreams
as hopes unfold magically

SUTRA 3

face your demons with compassion & bravery

You don't deserve to be here. You don't have what it takes. You are pretty for a dark-skinned girl. You look nothing like your mother. Your brother is so smart, but at least you can dance. Stop dreaming and focus. Wow, you are so articulate. They will see and hear all of your flaws. You are incapable of running the national department. You are too young. You haven't done this long enough. Wait your turn. She said you aren't ready to teach at these events. You need more years of experience. They will notice your inadequacies. No one wants to learn yoga from a black woman. Why are you so bossy? You are extremely selfish. Small businesses fail. Dreams don't come true. Get a real job. You don't have enough followers. Maybe you should show more skin in pictures. You aren't enough!

These are just some of the messages and thoughts that occupied my mind from childhood to Flyhood. I don't blame the emotional programming I received from my mother, father, and other adults in my life. My parents did the best they could; however, the signals definitely got crossed in my mind when their support of my extracurricular activities didn't match the verbal statements and secret conversations I overheard. About 60 percent of the time their words were more encouraging than limiting, but that other 40 percent consisted of negative words or actions that played out in the form of control, guilt, or shame. During therapy sessions in my thirties I realized my parents were great at supporting me when I excelled but horrible with encouraging and uplifting messages when I wasn't the absolute best, especially in school. The feelings wrapped around the words that they and my teachers and other adults used remained attached to my heart and clouded my decisions. When coworkers, friends, and even intimate partners tossed up negativity, it stuck, and I often reacted. Mostly, I would shrink, obsess for days, and sometimes use the negativity to prove them wrong. I basically dropped into old familiar patterns and allowed my personal demons to control my actions and life choices.

DEMONS IN THE DARK

Now that you have a taste of my childhood and a tiny glimpse into my rebirth, let's dive into the shadows. Let's talk about the demons lurking in the closet, and the evil inner voices saturating the depths of our DNA, occupying our thoughts, and paralyzing our actions. These devilish beings spill toxins into our headspace, firmly lock into our shoulders, and root into our hips, creating physical blockages. Their mystical powers manifest into varying levels of physical discomfort and push us headfirst into the fires of self-loathing. The crazy part is that we know these demons hold us back from living our "best life," but somehow our fear keeps us under their control.

You may have heard the phrase "shadow work." This is definitely a buzz concept within the self-help arena, and many spiritual teachers, healers, and therapists integrate these teachings into their practices. Before we approach facing your demons, it's important to understand this theory. Your shadow is the dark aspect of your personality that plays on the grounds of human emotions such as shame, envy, rage, anger, and greed, but also includes wants, desires, and the need for power. As young children we feel and experience all human emotions. Rays of light (love, tenderness, kindness, and compassion) balance effortlessly with the cast of shadow emotions. Through adult programming, we shift and morph by example and discipline. No, acting out and kicking my brothers wasn't the proper way to express my anger; however, repressing my anger and feeling a sense of shame for my feelings wasn't the best way to live through my teenage years either.

Over time we master the skill of hiding and disowning our shadow. We learn to suppress that side of ourselves and cloak our emotions with dysfunctional behavior. As a result, we sabotage relationships and careers, but mostly we sabotage our soul. The repression of these feelings can linger in our unconscious for years if we don't reconnect and become friends with them. The disowned shadow can even begin to dim our light.

Another way this plays out is through projection, which involves expressing anger, jealousy, envy, or other emotions toward someone else because we have repressed an aspect of their essence within ourselves. The process happens unconsciously and often we are completely unaware of our behavior. A few days before writing this section one of my staff refused to do their job because a client had "pushed her buttons." The client contacted me because she had been waiting on her materials for weeks. I spoke with the staff person, and she was so upset over the client that she quickly reacted to my request by saying, "No, Faith, you handle it." I paused, took a deep breath, and responded with a neutral, calm, nonjudgmental, yet firm statement of how our job is to deliver quality services regardless of the client's tone in emails. In that moment, I realized it was my employee's shadow coming through. Something had triggered her, and I knew that the best way to handle it was with a neutral and assertive directive. Days later the client received the materials, and I feel certain my employee took time to reflect on her actions.

Our unconscious shadow drops in swiftly and layers our thoughts with unhealthy egoic responses. In those split seconds we don't have time to autocorrect, and if we don't catch it post-reaction, self-assess, and work on recalibrating our subconscious, the mind will continue to ride old patterns and spiral inward to reaffirm the story, and then the cycle repeats itself. The really frightening part is when the unhealthy mind makes toxic decisions that burn your relationship bridges or career and pollute every part of your life. It's so scary when the demons drive all that you do, and you've taken on a victim mentality completely lacking in hope and optimism. Yes, the damage is done, but you are not trapped.

WORKING WITH THE DEMONS

I'm constantly making nice with the two-headed monster that has one head in the real world and one dancing in unconscious trickery. It's a crazy flow of recalibrating, resetting, and remembering my own spiritual brilliance. In order to live more fully in this human existence, we must wrap our arms around the cloudy shadow and see the monster as beautiful. We have to see the emotional demons as what makes us whole, and use them to make conscious choices based on our highest self. There's no time to baby your emotions; it's time to get dirty and extract what you have kept hidden for a lifetime. Like you and tons of others, I engaged in spiritual bypassing. I honestly thought my yoga and meditation practices made me a better person and that they would keep me in a state of "love and light." They didn't! Let me say it a different way: getting on your yoga mat every day and feeling juicy in the flow is *not* going to save your soul. Yoga, meditation, ayahuasca, and many other spiritual practices only cradle the spirit and make us feel held. And no, going to church every Sunday will not save you either. All are beautiful methods of personal elevation, but as complex humans, we have to utilize an assortment of tools to recalibrate our minds and rewire our hearts. So here we go. Let's drop in and do the "monster mash."

RECALIBRATE MEDITATION & JOURNALING

This is a very intense and sometimes emotionally draining exercise. At the same time, it has the ability to support massive shift and additional self-discovery. Grab a pen and paper and give yourself at least thirty to forty-five minutes for this exercise.

JOURNALING

In a seated position, take five to seven deep breaths and then answer these questions as honestly as you can.

- Who do you strongly dislike?
- Make a list of the behaviors, physical characteristics, and achievements that bother you about this individual or this type of person.

- Are there multiple people in your life with these characteristics and behaviors?
- How do you see these qualities reflected in yourself?
- How have you disowned or suppressed this aspect of yourself?

MEDITATION

Select one behavior or characteristic to work with during this meditation. Set your timer for ten minutes. Lie down on your back and place your palms on the sacral area of your body (slightly below your navel). Imagine your inner self rising from your physical body and opening the door to your room. As you go through the door, begin to walk along a golden path that leads to your favorite place in nature. Feel your feet grounded beneath you and

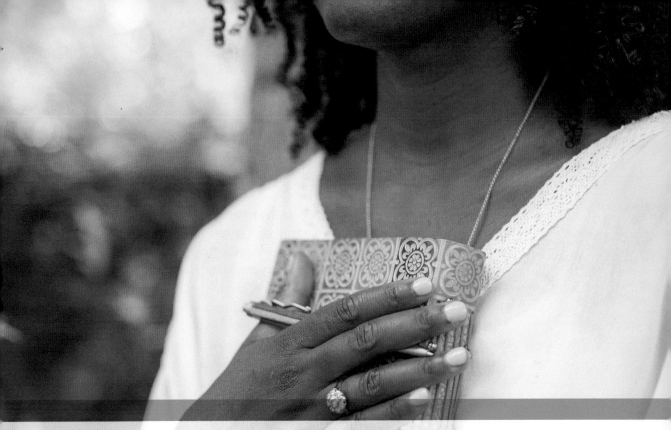

a sense of safety, security, and stability. Once you feel this, begin to think about a time during childhood where you saw the selected behavior or characteristic in yourself or someone else. See how this behavior or characteristic was shamed or criticized. Take note of your age, and who did the shaming or criticizing. Now begin to shift the story of this situation by letting go of the shame, fear, and uncomfortable thoughts. If your parents or another adult caused the negative thoughts, visualize how they could have approached the situation differently. If it was another child, use your voice by speaking up. For example, if I was shamed for the color of my skin, I could visualize myself speaking up and saying, "I love my skin and being the color of dark chocolate." Once you have recalibrated the story, remain still for a few more minutes, then slowly begin to bring yourself out of the meditative state.

JOURNALING

Write down whatever came up during the meditation. Describe the shift in the story. How did you feel after the shift and prior to coming out of the meditation?

Note: I recommend working on each behavior or characteristic individually until you no longer disown it within yourself, and you are no longer looking down on others for exhibiting it. It could take weeks to months, so give yourself time to transform these patterns. Repeat the meditation at least two to three time a week while your subconscious is shifting.

DANCING IN THE SHADOWS

I know the exercise above was hard, but you have to give yourself a break. Thousands of thoughts dance across the stage of our mind every single second, and it's impossible for us to control all of them. The subconscious moves these thoughts in and out, and when we see and experience something in the moment that triggers a past experience, we bring feelings from that time forward. We respond to what's directly in front of us, and energetically recall the past. That's why the previous exercise is so important. The work is about reprogramming the subconscious. Even if we haven't experienced a situation before, our intuition guides us through the process of responding based on a similar experience from the past. And when our past is rooted in shame and fear, we are more likely to engage negative sensations and entertain negative thoughts on a really powerful level. I keep coming back to this work because it intimately impacts the way we move and navigate adulthood. When we don't address these thoughts and feelings through deep spiritual work and are unable to catch ourselves reacting in the present moment, we create stories around what we could or should do.

When we move honestly into self-awareness, we are able to wrap compassion around fear and shame. Compassion requires us to care, to be empathetic, sympathetic, and nonjudgmental, and to have a deep level of understanding when things are really uncomfortable. But compassion is also filled with positive emotions like joy, contentment, bliss, optimism, human connection, and overall personal satisfaction. In our self-deprecating mind filled with inadequacies, it's hard to have compassion for ourselves and others. I believe the first step to self-compassion is finding your center; however, there's not a single center. I often laugh when I hear myself and other yoga teachers say, "Find your center." There are actually four centers within each human, and

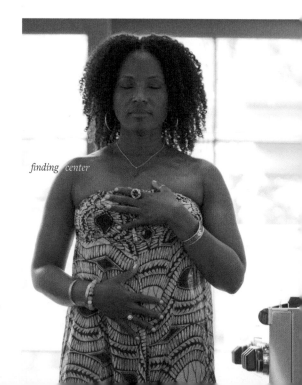

finding center

they have been brilliantly discussed within Hinduism, Taoism, and other ancient philosophies. These centers are as follows:

- Physical: located below the navel
- Emotional: located around the center of the chest
- Mental: located around and at the center of the brain
- Spiritual: floats above the crown of the head

Finding your center is one of the most useful tools for dancing with the demons in the present moment. It gives you the ability to slow down, process your feelings, and avoid pushing more negativity through your mind and projecting it onto someone else. So when you are in a challenging situation, or when you hear a yoga teacher say, "Find your center," think about how you can mindfully notice the sensations of the physical body, access your emotional state, steady the mind so you direct it into the current moment, and align to the sacredness of your highest self. It seems really difficult, but in those moments you are truly dancing center stage with your demon.

I must say, the following exercise is one of the only ways I can fully reconnect with my center on the fly. Meditation definitely helps as a long-term strategy, but what if you only have thirty seconds? What if you are in the middle of several triggers? How can you pull yourself out of the spiral? How can you find your center?

THIRTY SECONDS TO CENTER

Make this technique your go-to tool whenever and wherever you need to. When you feel yourself being triggered negatively by your shadow, do the following:

- STOP! Gaze at one spot and begin to take slow deep breaths (this will slow down your heart rate).
- Bring awareness to your feet, legs, hands, arms, and torso.
- Notice your emotions, and what you are feeling from your heart.
- Continue to breathe and allow your mind to focus only on the breath.
- Then begin to imagine sending energy from the soles of the feet to the crown of your head.
- Once you direct your energy to the crown, take a big inhale and then slowly exhale out of the mouth.
- If you have time, repeat the steps, moving through each phase slowly.

THE DEMON OF SHAME

Another aspect of facing your shadow demons is releasing shame and then using that subconscious break to amplify what I like to call your "Golden Glitter." First let's talk about shame, then I'll drop my definition of Golden Glitter. Shame is directly attached to self-worth. Self-worth is very different from self-esteem for it goes beyond the highest feeling of your value; it's deeply knowing and personally recognizing your greatness.

From birth to adulthood, we regulate our behavior based on external responses, and our self-worth is created through imprints on the mind made by our experiences. For example, when we express ourselves as children, we are either praised or punished, and the behavior is placed in a category of good or bad. In addition, we observe the behavior and actions of others and notice the reactions they receive from our parents/caretakers, other adults, and even classmates. What we perceive as bad or negative takes shape in the subconscious and unfolds in the form of shame when we behave or engage in that manner. Yes, it all comes back to family, friends, and media. I'm not casting blame; I'm simply identifying why we respond in certain ways and make the choices about our lives that we do. Facing the shame reveals a clear picture of our patterns and gives us the strength to move in a direction based on our own beliefs and values. It also creates an emotional foundation for personal growth.

Golden Glitter is made up of the magical particles of self-worth that are sprinkled across and throughout every area of your life, and like real glitter, it's almost impossible to get rid of. When you know who you are and feel comfortable enough to be yourself in all settings, your Golden Glitter is felt through dialogue, absorbed by others through eye contact, and left behind in their hearts and memories. When you recognize your personal strengths, talents, and passions and allow them to inspire your career, the universe cocreates through opportunities and easy personal manifestation. Oprah's Golden Glitter is insanely bright and magnified and can be experienced, felt, and absorbed like a glitter bomb. The power of her Golden Glitter is transferred across the media and replayed by millions of people every day. Now if you are thinking you could never reach that state, pause and do the "Thirty Seconds to Center" scan you practiced above. Notice what comes up; it's definitely a little demon lingering from childhood. It's simply a subconscious experience that attempted to wash away your Golden Glitter or dim its radiance.

FACING SHAME MEDITATION & JOURNALING

This exercise, like the previous one, might bring up lots of old stuff. Be kind, don't judge yourself, and do not—DO NOT—wrap more shame around what comes up. Give yourself about fifteen to thirty minutes.

CENTERING MEDITATION

Take five to ten minutes to center before the journaling session. Find a private space where you feel safe and comfortable. Grab your journal or a piece of paper. Sit comfortably on the floor or in a chair. Close your eyes and begin to take slow, deep breaths. As you breathe, walk through the steps you did in the "Thirty Seconds to Center" exercise but instead take at least five to ten minutes. Take your time to feel and become fully aware of your physical, emotional, mental, and spiritual centers.

JOURNALING

The next few questions will require you to acknowledge and physically write down your demons. If some of them are too difficult to deal with now, don't worry. You can always focus on just one question at a time. Remember, this process could take days or months, so dealing with one issue at a time is totally appropriate. If you can handle all four questions, go for it. I recommend doing this over the course of a month and revisiting each question two to five times.

Always do the meditation prior to answering a question. As you work through this exercise, different situations may start to come up, and you may begin to remember more than you anticipated. Don't worry; your mind is simply unclogging, clearing, and making space.

Note: At the end of each question, close your eyes for five minutes. During this time I want you to release and reset any emotional shame attached to the past experience. Visualize how your heart and soul wanted to respond. Feel it, believe it, and reset.

• What moment or situation in your early childhood (up to twelve years old) created a sense of shame? Was this part of your parents'/guardians' response to you? Did you see one of them project shame or levels of negativity toward each other or someone else? How has this impacted your adult experiences and decisions with friends, family, work, intimate relationships, and so on? How has it shaped your view of self? Meditate and reset this in your subconscious.

• In your teen years, what decisions did you make that you felt were judged by your peers or the adults in your life? When others make similar decisions, do you cast judgment? When it bubbles up in your mind, does shame immediately surface? Meditate and reset this in your subconscious.

- List the people you have betrayed or who betrayed you. Did an apology happen on either side? How did you feel after the apology? Meditate and reset this in your subconscious.

As we know, Oprah has done and continues to do a significant amount of deep personal and spiritual work, which allows her to shine and sprinkle her Golden Glitter on others. My own evolution has birthed the tips, techniques, and practices that I share in this book, and it's rooted in knowing that when I'm being held hostage by my own mind, my heart and soul cannot elevate. So when the demon of shame casts darkness over my decisions through the second-guessing of my intuition or the fear of what others might think, it's time for me to face shame with a little compassionate force.

Childhood stories are filled with evil demons focused on controlling, capturing, and ultimately possessing. Because we have these impressions we think have been set, we convince ourselves that we can't be more than we already are. I knew I had a natural gift as a ballet dancer, and I witnessed the unfolding of greatness throughout my childhood. That included affirmations from my parents and other adults. On the other hand, reading was a challenge in school, and I was shamed by my parents and other adults because I wasn't as "smart" as my brothers. Even now, I sometimes drop into my insecure headspace. When it starts to rise, I have to pause, breathe, and reset with a positive visualization of those moments in childhood and adulthood when I excelled because of my mind. Negative thoughts are reshaped by positive messages, which stimulate the flow of energy so I can crawl out. Knowing and valuing my worth around my mental capacity is simply one example in my life where shame impacted my choices and decisions and often played out in my relationships. Basically the subconscious pulls the feeling from the past and projects it into the present, and then we react in an effort to fit in and be normal. The real work happens by becoming aware, identifying the backstories of the demons, and resetting the feeling that lives in the mind.

RELEASING THE ANGER

During the periods of looking at my shadow and facing the demons, anger always rises to the top. I never know when it will happen, but I never stop the feeling. A fellow yoga teacher asked me a few months ago if I get angry. I, of course, responded with a yes. She went on to share that she feels guilty when anger starts to rumble in her heart, especially when she's upset in a relationship or frustrated with herself for getting angry. Then when she drops into a love and kindness meditation, it sometimes gets even worse. I shared that anger is the result of another feeling or emotion that we haven't dealt with, and when that is repeated over and over and never addressed, our mind sends a signal telling us to get angry. For instance, if we feel afraid, disrespected, trapped, or even pressured, our mind starts to express that in the form of anger. In our culture, especially the "yoga culture," we avoid the underlying emotions, feel the anger rise, and then suppress it along with the other emotions. We are handing ourselves a double dose of "spiritual bypassing." We are avoiding all feelings, emotions, and shadows in an effort to feel good.

Culturally this is also linked to adults encouraging children to be "good little girls and boys." Then as adults, we jump into yoga and meditation classes seeking that sweet spot of *ananda*, which in Sanskrit means "bliss" or "divine joy." Then at some point in the midst of our crazy life, we experience a taste of the yummy deliciousness of ananda on a random day during class. Like a "yoga addict," we keep chasing that high and assuming that if we let go of our anger, ananda is ours to keep and life will be perfect. Some people will forever do this dance and wonder why they are still filled with guilt, shame, and overall dysfunction. I believe part of the demon dance is addressing our shadow and being okay with getting angry about why it's there. If we never feel the feeling and get angry, it sits and clogs our physical, emotional, mental, and spiritual centers. Anger is a real human emotion, and it's okay to feel it, but it's even more important to be self-aware and know why it's present. So when I am overwhelmed with anger, I first breathe and ask myself, why? If the spin cycle is out of control, I plug into the following "Fists of Anger" exercise.

KUNDALINI MEDITATION: FISTS OF ANGER

This is a meditation for releasing anger by channeling the energy and opening the portals through breath and movement.

HOW TO PRACTICE   Come into a comfortable seated position and tune in with *Ong Namo Guru Dev Namo*. Make a fist with both hands by first touching the tips of your thumbs to the bases of your pinky fingers and then wrapping your other fingers over your thumbs. Lift your arms up and over your head and, one at a time, swing them in a backstroke movement, alternating right and left.

As you continue to swing your arms, close your eyes and breathe in and out through an O-shaped mouth in rhythm with your arm swings. Do this for three minutes. At the same time, think about what made you angry and the underlying reason it did. If others issues of anger start coming up, it's okay. Stay with the practice, increasing the movement and breath.

To end, interlace your fingers and extend your arms overhead, pressing your palms toward the sky. Inhale through an O-shaped mouth and imagine yourself surrounded by healing white light. Hold for a few seconds, then exhale through an O-shaped mouth. Repeat this three times.

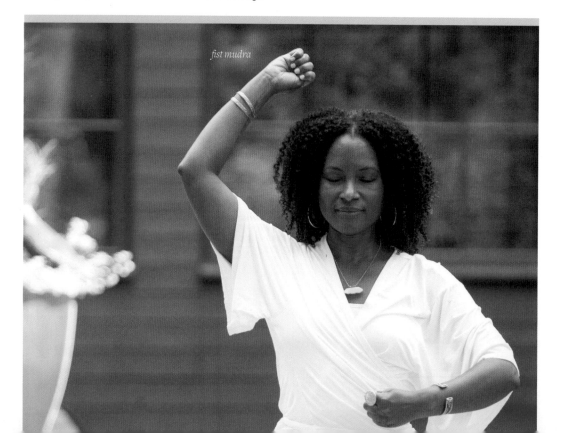

fist mudra

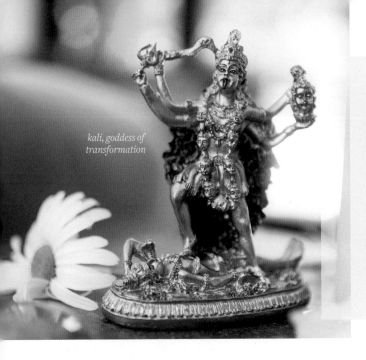

kali, goddess of transformation

Slay the Demons: A Poem to Kali

release all that is not free
may your waves of compassion purify my soul
destroy the unreal
elevate my transcendental breath
so I may
be brave and fierce to taste the
    flavors of the world
dance among cycles of karma
and triple my awareness
past present future

When I think about slaying demons, my mind immediately jumps to the Hindu goddess Kali. She's mentioned in association with death and violence, but I soak up the perspective of bravely supporting us with motherly love. As the destroyer and slayer of evil forces, she energetically grants *moksha*, or liberation, by removing the illusions of the ego. The garland of skulls around her neck and the skirt of dismembered arms she wears represent our identification with the body. We are caught up in the cycle of shame and fear, and our illusions of this are demonstrated by our actions and choices. Through sacred practices, we have the capacity to call upon our inner Kali and free ourselves from mental trappings. With her eyes blazing wide and hands holding severed heads dripping in blood, I feel Kali represents the eternal battle we have with ourselves. Struggling with the negativity, yet winning with consistent practice and dedication.

So now I want you to embrace your inner Kali and disconnect those actions, shame, and pain that are keeping you from letting your Golden Glitter shine. As I shared earlier, our brains associate the actions of shame with self-worth and self-esteem. When these emotional attachments latch onto our soul, their energy drags us down and often causes us to repeat the actions in a similar form. Here's the deal: once you bring them to the surface with self-awareness and reset the subconscious, you have to chop off their heads. You don't need get all crazy and obsessed about them; just get in there and slay the little monsters. Visualization and meditation are two tools that can help, but know that some of these demons are vicious. Their strength and emotional heaviness dims our light and darkens our aura. I've seen

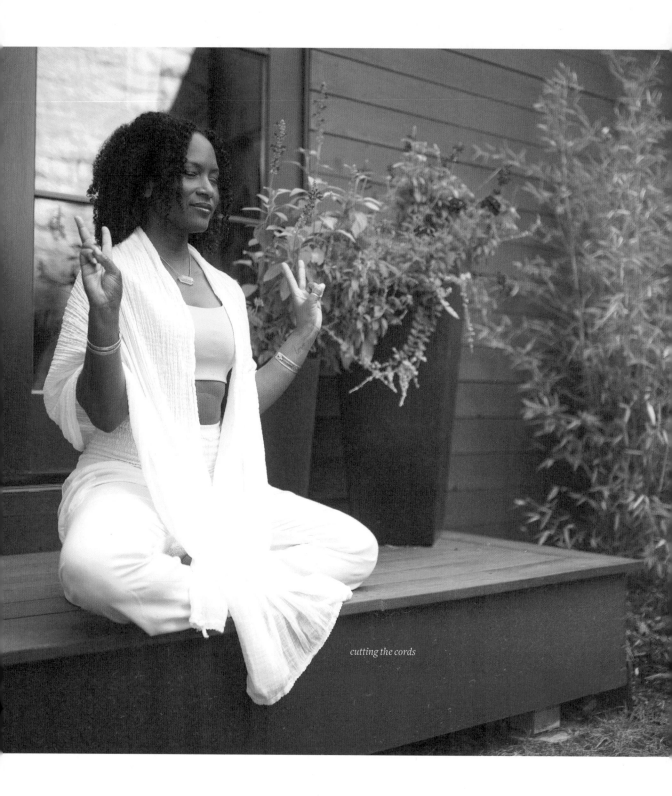

cutting the cords

this happen within myself and watched it play out in intimate relationships. Even when I think I've done the work, I unconsciously drop back into my old patterns. It's a bizarre flow of energy that can easily hide in the shadows and creep into daily life, causing dysfunction when we least expect it. That's what makes the personal work so powerful, and why it's essential to maintain a daily practice as a foundation and utilize targeted practices to cut through the serious bullshit we tell ourselves.

CUTTING THE CORDS

One of the most effective targeted practices I use after the "Working with Demons" exercises is called "Cutting the Cords." This practice helps to slay the haunting toxic energy of shame, fear, unproductive habits, other people, and situations that constantly pops up, and works to release it from your soul. It's not a daily practice, but it's a great exercise to have in your emotional toolbox.

HOW TO PRACTICE   Come into a comfortable seated position and close your eyes. Allow your breath to flow smoothly in and out of your nose. Do this for about one to two minutes. Begin to imagine yourself glowing in your highest place of divinity, holding golden, glitter-covered Kali swords. Allow that strength to rush through each center (physical, emotional, mental, and spiritual). Know you have the inner fortitude to cut the negative messaging,

shame, fear, pain, and discomfort that are dimming your light.

Once you feel ready, lift both arms so your hands are at shoulder height. Bend your elbows and let them rest near your body. Extend your index and middle fingers. These are your swords. Your thumbs hold down your ring and little fingers. Begin to open and close your extended fingers and as you do so, visually see yourself slaying the demons with ease. Imagine them detaching from center. Do this for two to five minutes.

When you feel complete, raise both arms over your head in a *V* shape and spread your fingers wide. Hold your breath for five seconds, then repeat two more times. As you exhale each time, repeat this mantra: *release you from my soul.* Bring your hands to rest on your thighs and sit in stillness for at least one minute. Then slowly open your eyes.

This simple technique enables us to soften the spirit and wraps a beautiful, compassionate blanket around the soul. It can be done at any time of the day. I strongly encourage you to do it for at least twenty-one days. As the days go by, you will notice that fewer demons surface and your mind grows more calm.

yoga practice
facing your demons

As you work through the following exercises and meditations, you will feel tons of emotions bubble to the top, you will connect deeper to your sense of self-worth, and without a doubt, you will experience moments of inner freedom. Throughout the slaying-demons process I recommend doing these three postures to support you in building physical and emotional stamina. You're free to do these separately when you need an energetic lift, or merge them into your own personal yoga practice.

mantra
I am a brave warrior.

PLANK POSE (*PHALAKASANA*)   With no other choice but to feel, this posture draws upon the core to maintain physical stability. When the abdomen is engaged, we stimulate the third chakra (solar plexus). This chakra is related to confidence, willpower, and the perception of who you are at the "core." Plank Pose also strengthens and tones the chest, shoulders, arms, wrists, and lower back and aids in toning the nervous system. It is one of postures repeated in a Sun Salutation or during a flow, but it is also perfect as a standalone.

HOW TO PRACTICE   Come onto all fours with your wrists under your shoulders. Spread your fingers wide with your middle fingers pointing forward. As your hands press into the floor, ensure that your weight is distributed throughout and that you aren't placing pressure on the heels of your hands. If you have wrist issues, come to your forearms with your elbows aligned with your shoulders. Draw your lower belly in toward your spine and up toward your ribs. Stay here or extend your legs behind with your toes tucked. As you create a straight line with your body, keep your thighs engaged and extend your tailbone toward your heels. Firmly draw your triceps together and keeping your arms in the beginning position, slide your shoulder blades down and along your spine and press them toward the ceiling. Press away from the floor and gaze slightly past your fingertips. Hold the posture for five to ten breaths and repeat three to five times, taking short ten- to fifteen-second breaks. At the end, relax on the belly and rest for one minute.

KUNDALINI ARCHER POSE Very similar in form to Warrior II, this posture grounds us in our earthly reality, develops keen focus, and improves personal awareness. As it builds physical stamina by strengthening the legs, ankles, and feet, the posture also stretches the legs, ankles, groin, chest, lungs, and shoulders. On a lovely energetic level, it softens tension within the heart and strengthens one's aura, which creates a powerful presence. Simply stated, it's a Golden Glitter amplifier.

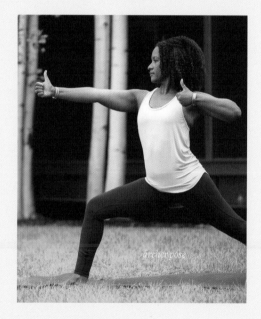

archer pose

HOW TO PRACTICE   Standing with feet parallel, step your right foot back (three to four feet, depending on the length of your legs and the openness of your hips). Point the toes of your left foot toward the top of the mat and place your right foot at a 90-degree angle. The heel or inner arch of your right foot is aligned with the heel of your left foot. If you feel unstable, bring your aligned heels farther apart. Breathe in and as you exhale, slowly bend your left knee so it stacks over your left ankle. If it doesn't go all the way, don't push it. Also, don't go past your ankle. Spread your toes wide and firmly press into both feet to create more stability. Lift your arms parallel to the floor and bring both hands into fists. Bend your right elbow, keeping your upper right arm parallel to the ground. Your right elbow points back and your right hand is at your chest, making a gesture of pulling a bow and arrow. Extend the thumb of the left hand and gaze at it with the spirit of a warrior. Start out holding this posture for thirty seconds and build your way up to five minutes. Take long, deep breaths the entire time. Repeat on the other side.

SKULL SHINING BREATH (*KAPALABHATI*)   *Kapalabhati*—from *kapala* meaning "skull" and *bhati* meaning "light"—is a detoxing technique that purifies both physically and mentally. In the state of activation, it rejuvenates, invigorates, cuts through sluggishness, and helps to relieve stress. When I watch my students do this breathing practice, I can immediately see the energy shift within them.

HOW TO PRACTICE   Sit comfortably with your spine straight and your hands resting on your thighs. Take three to four deep breaths through your nose. Inhale to a comfortable level (about half way) and then exhale sharply, forcefully pushing the air out through the nose, while at the same time contracting the belly as you exhale. Allow the inhale to happen passively. Continue forcefully exhaling and passively inhaling at a steady and powerful pace. The belly is pumping continuously, and the movement is coming from the diaphragm. Do this for one minute. Pause for ten to twenty seconds and repeat two more times. Between sets, come back to deep inhales and exhales. At the end, return to a balanced breathing pattern and be in stillness for two to three minutes. If you feel lightheaded at any time, return to slow inhales and exhales. If you are pregnant, have just given birth, or on the first few days of your moon cycle, don't practice this technique. Also, be mindful if you have high blood pressure, asthma, emphysema, or a heart condition.

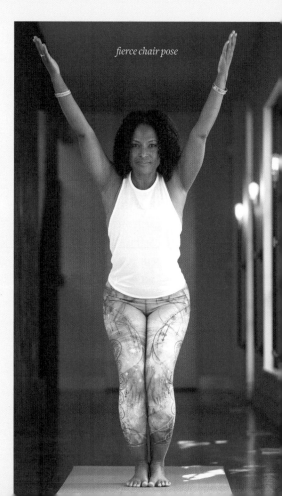

fierce chair pose

FIERCE CHAIR POSE (*UTKATASANA*) WITH SKULL SHINING BREATH (*KAPALABHATI*)   When I first started teaching my Spiritually Fly yoga classes, Chair Pose was a staple. It worked perfectly because *utkata* means "fierce, proud, immense, and large"—all of the qualities that activate and support self-worth. The bend in the knees drops the hips and creates a grounding sensation that strengthens the feet, ankles, and thighs. At the same time it tones the butt, hips, shoulders, and back muscles. Having the arms overhead directs the energy upward, opens the chest, increases the heart rate, and stimulates the digestive organs and the circulatory and metabolic systems.

HOW TO PRACTICE FIERCE CHAIR POSE   Stand with your feet parallel, hip-bone distance apart, with the weight balanced between both feet. Breathe in, and on the exhale bend your knees and reach your hips back so your weight shifts behind you without lifting the balls of your feet. It's like you are about to sit in a chair. Keep your upper body leaning slightly forward and keep your chest open. Once you feel steady, slowly lift your arms overhead with the palms facing inward. You are also welcome to bring the palms together overhead, but only if you can keep your shoulders relaxed. If you have a shoulder injury, bring your palms together at your heart or keep them next to your hips. Draw your shoulders down and away from your ears, gaze straight ahead, and engage your abdominal muscles while directing the sitz bones toward the floor. Hold the posture for five breaths, then repeat two more times.

HOW TO PRACTICE FIERCE CHAIR POSE WITH KAPALABHATI   Come into Fierce Chair Pose slowly and mindfully. Take one to two breaths in the posture and begin one minute of Kapalabhati breath, keeping your eyes focused on a single point. At the end, slowly stand and return to a natural breathing pattern for three to five breaths. Repeat two more times. Once all three repetitions are complete, stand with your feet slightly apart, close your eyes, and observe the physical and mental sensations. Simply notice and feel.

KUNDALINI MEDITATION: REMOVING FEAR OF THE FUTURE

When cultivating compassion for and bravery with our demons, it's essential to engage in a twenty-one-day meditation. This meditation is perfect for removing the fear that's sitting in our subconscious memories of the past. As it connects to the flow of the heart center, fear is released. I suggest making this an evening meditation practice.

HOW TO PRACTICE   Sit in a comfortable cross-legged position. You can also straighten the legs while sitting on the floor, or sit in a chair. Tune in by chanting *Ong Namo Guru Dev Namo* three times. Place the left hand in the palm of the right hand. Wrap the right hand around the left hand with the right thumb nestled in the left palm, and the fingers holding gently around the left hand. Place the hands against the heart center (center of the chest).

Play the *Dhan Dhan Ram Das Gur* mantra (there are many versions online; find the one that resonates with you) while meditating for eleven minutes and slowly work your way up to thirty-one minutes. Close the meditation with an extended *Sat Nam*.

As humans, we are forever shifting, transforming, and developing. In utero through infancy we absorb a significant amount of energy from our mother and other individuals around us. Although communication is limited, we are mostly a sponge to be held, protected, loved, and nurtured. Once we rise into our toddler phase, our exploration expands, and we test our limits. By the time we enter childhood (ages five to eleven), we begin to make decisions based on prior experiences, and we learn that our actions have consequences. This is also when we begin to develop a sense of self. With the hormone-infused body of adolescence, our thoughts and actions are about identity and personal expressions. Regardless of one's childhood, adolescence can be scary, confusing, and emotionally draining. If we didn't receive love, safety, support, understanding, and nurturing from infancy to eleven years old, we are definitely on the prowl for them now. That means in adulthood, we are still chasing those qualities, but they are now living in the form of old patterns and behaviors. They are showing up as demons—responding, reacting, and creating a nightmare in your life.

the source of divine transformation is within.

In order to live the life you desire and be able to revel in your Golden Glitter, you have to do the work. You have to craft time to recalibrate your physical, emotional, mental, and spiritual centers. It takes more than one feel-good moment or technique. This Spiritually Fly life is about using a combination of tools and practices to dance with your demons. The process will be uncomfortable and at times super scary. The journaling and meditations will bring up lots of old shit and years of suppressed memories. Fortunately, this approach of merging physical movement, intentional techniques, and personal commitment gives you the capacity and strength to face your demons. When the anger dips in, see it and feel it and know that you have the stamina to bravely move with it. When sadness washes over you, allow your heart to comfort the emotions and nurture yourself with ultimate compassion.

This deep spiritual work of facing your demons requires you to peel back layers of old habits and be brave enough to release the heavily ingrained behaviors. In the fog of the uncomfortable, you will begin to design something more authentic; you will see the light of your soul that you thought was lost. With this clear understanding of your value and worth, and a healthy relationship with your demons, you will gracefully elevate into your highest self.

each moment I show up
a modern ritual of breathing,
   reflecting, and refining
not just my physical body
but the deepest realms of
   my eternal existence
this is more than just a practice
this is my life
a powerful connection to myself,
   others, and the divine
fearlessly unraveling the knots
with the highest desire to stay present
I drop into a place where my soul swoons
and my body realigns
this is my yoga, my dharma, my path
this is what I call spiritually flying

let your walls down, reveal your heart

rolling over to the sound of snores and the feel of body heat, my mind returned to Jake again. I opened my eyes and there he was: the gorgeous Italian man I had met in a DC club. Within a few weeks we were an item. Within a year I relocated to New York City to be closer to him and figure out what I really wanted out of life. Unsure of my true passions, I floated around Manhattan in the summer of 2001 hunting for a job, practicing lots of yoga, discovering all that the city had to offer, and cohabiting with a kind partner. Life was sweet, but somehow I was still unhappy. My mind danced around my own insecurities. I secretly doubted myself at every turn and constantly wondered if Jake was really the man for me. The insecure thoughts were compounded by 9/11, and by November 17, 2001 my father had died. My heart was heavy, I cried constantly, and I built a stone wall around my heart.

As I lay in bed on an unsettling night, my anxiety kicked in to overdrive, and I was in a state of obsession. I felt extremely disconnected, alone, and sad. All I could think about was not having a strong and grounding masculine force in my life. By then, my father and older brother were dead, and I didn't have a deep connection with anyone, male or female, including Jake. I cowardly ended the relationship, and within weeks I jumped back into the dating pool. Not to have a boyfriend, but simply just to hang. I avoided the emotional river of deep intimacy, and I only dated guys who desired zero commitment. When things started to get serious, I would ghost or abruptly end the relationship. Real talk: I was a honeymoon master and a breakup queen.

Within the dysfunction of my own behavior, I cried most nights. My level of depression increased, and I decided to see a therapist. The weekly therapy sessions unpacked my childhood relationship with my father and discovered how the fear of abandonment created a wall years before I was old enough to date. Basically, my father's Army career kept him away from us because my parents felt we needed a permanent home environment surrounded by other family members. As a result, my father was always leaving. Watching him come and go created the fear of being abandoned, but it was also one of my shadows around feeling worthy and having love, even for myself. Therapy helped me see my patterns, access my behavior, and develop tools of connecting differently to myself and others.

WEIGHT OF THE HEART

The human heart weighs eight to twelve ounces depending on the size of the body. This seems super light in comparison to how we feel after a death, divorce, trauma (physical and emotional), or loss of something we have become emotionally attached to through experiences translated into joyous memories. Because we will no longer engage in life, playing in the grassy fields of these moments, our mind and body drop into sensations of heaviness. With the heaviness comes sadness, and in the sadness we begin to hide and shelter our hearts. There are an assortment of reasons why the walls are built, but it's impossible to be in the fullness of life behind the walls.

Sadness and a heavy heart are basic human emotions we all experience. If the sad moments are not dealt with in a healthy manner, the mind starts to draw lines around the heart in preparation for constructing a wall. Once the wall is built, it takes intentional explosives and "soul fire" to knock it down. Soul fire is a way of unpacking, burning, and purifying old patterns and unresolved emotions so a new foundation can be poured, and you can start again. Many of my clients have asked my advice around love and have wanted help in mending a broken heart. I found that it didn't matter what type of love they had lost or in what context, the grief was part of what we all feel in the valley of love. When the fire burns down the wall, love in all forms can be regained.

In an effort to stop feeling pain and sadness after the loss of her mother, one of my clients isolated herself from the rest of her family and pulled away from her friends. She knew distancing herself from the people she loved wasn't the answer, but she simply didn't want to be reminded of the pain. In addition, she didn't want to create new memories, especially with her nieces and nephews. This emotional detachment created more separation, and she started to pull away from friends. After a night of sobbing, she decided to find a meditation online. Somewhere between searching for a meditation and more crying, she came across my story of loss. It resonated with her, and she reached out. At the time I was still doing private sessions, and we connected in person. Over the course of three months, we worked together weekly and upon my recommendation, she saw a therapist as well.

We can't avoid pain and sadness, and we definitely can't hide and hope that pain does not find us. The beauty of being human is feeling the heaviness, understanding it from an emotional level, and experiencing the memories of grief and joy with openness. But the balance is being okay and brave enough to connect, feel hope, and run fiercely in the fields of intimacy.

CRACKS IN THE WALLS

The magnificence of our hearts is more expansive than we can imagine. We have a capacity to love passionately, give in a million ways, celebrate in various forms, and express the internal elevations of the heart that's greater than any other species on earth. Our souls are woven to connect and naturally rest in a place of openness. And with a simple touch, glance, or presence, we can experience and share the magical vibration of love across cultures. Because we are emotional beings with sensitive hearts, it's okay to go slow and easy when we start to dismantle the walls. And the way we do that is by making tiny cracks to weaken the structure. Here are a few examples:

- Be open to the possibility that your heart's walls can crumble. When my student realized in the comfort of her own home that something had to change, she figured online meditation was a good place to start. She could have easily picked up the phone and called a family member, but it would have been too much for her emotionally. Instead, she opened to no longer feeling sad. She created a crack by taking steps to feel more secure within herself, and seeing the possibility of reconnecting with her family when she was ready.

- Find and learn ways of coping with loss. There's no way to avoid all the circumstances that can cause a heavy or broken heart, and the statement "just get over it" never works. It is, however, really important to gain tools and personalized techniques of coping with the experience. I always recommend more than one tool, and when someone has built a fortress, I suggest therapy or group counseling. Keep in mind that having an assortment of tools doesn't mean you avoid or suppress situations when they happen. The key is feeling and coping through the wave of emotions with supportive tools.

- Your heart is yours, so release emotional comparisons. Too often we place judgment around the speed at which others make it through the dark, or worse, we see that our ex is back in the dating game only a week after they broke up with us. Comparing your heart to another's will only block the process and create a stronger structure. This crack comes back to compassion and self-love. Don't be too hard on yourself, and believe in the path you are on. Mend, trust your intuition, and be okay with moving through your loss in your own time.

HEART AND SOUL

Along with weekly therapy, a daily meditation practice, yoga, and journaling, I slowly crawled out the hole, and glimmers of hope started to shine through. I began to clarify my meaning of joy and started to examine what it looked like for me. Around this same time, I decided to become a yoga teacher. The crazy part about the riveting events of 2001 and the toxic choices around dating in 2002 is that they guided me to the Laughing Lotus Yoga Center. Within the colorful walls and loud music, I danced, cried, and tasted the lightness of God at every turn. I reconnected to my joy, and I felt the beauty of love from the inside out. Hope seeped into my heart, and my soul melted into a place of ease.

ONE-MINUTE BREATH & JOURNALING YOUR SADNESS

As you move through and create tiny cracks in the walls around the heart, take time to journal your thoughts and feelings. This journaling exercise combined with One-Minute Breath is a loving and compassionate way to move in a direction of possibility and work on healing the pain. It's also a great method for acknowledging that you aren't your grief; it doesn't own you, and you can use it as a tool to build deeper intimacy with yourself and others. Before you begin journaling, practice One-Minute Breath for three minutes. At the end of the three minutes, sit in silence for as long as you wish, then answer the questions below.

ONE-MINUTE BREATH

This breathing technique helps to calm the nerves, reduces anxiety, and settles the mind when it's in a worried state. As it brings you into the present moment, the hemispheres of the brain are balanced and optimized. By sitting and breathing this twenty/twenty/twenty method, you heighten the connection between the right and left hemispheres of the brain, and you strengthen the glandular system (endocrine system). This system includes the pineal gland, pituitary gland, hypothalamus, thyroid, parathyroid, thymus, pancreas, adrenals, and ovaries/testes. When these glands are functioning properly, they produce hormones that relay crucial information in a rhythmic pulse, communicating vital healing information to the nervous system, brain, and other major glands. Basically this and many other meditations included in this book open a spiritual doorway to shifting a negative mindset that will in turn enable you to release patterns and live more vibrantly.

HOW TO PRACTICE   Sit comfortably (on the floor or in a chair). Set the timer for three minutes and close your eyes. Inhale for twenty seconds, hold the breath for twenty seconds, and exhale for twenty seconds. If this is challenging, start with five to ten seconds for each part, then move to fifteen seconds, and work your way up to twenty seconds. Do your best to keep all three parts the same. At the end of three minutes, sit silently in meditation for as long as it feels natural.

Note: This a great breathing practice to use when your mind is spinning, so I encourage you to practice it when you are in those moments of emotional imbalance. Feel free to work your way up to eleven minutes.

JOURNALING

Do this journaling exercise as a way to connect to your heart and navigate emotions. Complete the following statements based on how you feel today.

- Today I am having a hard time because . . .
- I miss my loved one because . . .
- It is hard to move forward when . . .
- When I feel grief, pain, or sadness, I do or say . . .
- I feel steady and more like myself when I . . .
- My support system includes . . .
- I am ready to feel . . .

The soul can be defined as the spiritual aspect of the being that gives life to the physical form, or the spirit of God that lives within the being as a reflection of the imperishable. In West Africa, the goddess N'Game is described as the African moon goddess of soul and the creatress filled with the divine feminine power and authority to give humans and animals their soul. She carries a crescent-shaped bow and lunar arrows coated with the gift of life. When she shoots into the heart, life is granted. It is believed that when the arrow goes in, part of her divine essence pours into the being in the form of *kra*, the soul that never dies. While the physical form may die, the soul lives on because it comes from N'Game, and it will return to earth in another form. N'Game is basically the mother and creatress of all things; she is life force, or prana, and the pulse of energy that runs through us.

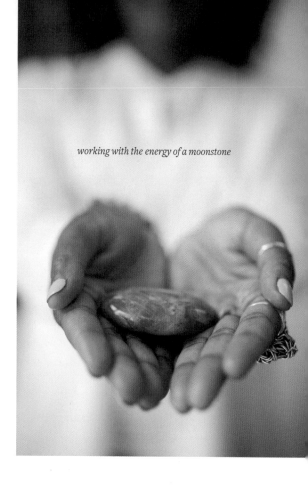

working with the energy of a moonstone

My soul may hide, but it will never die.

Inspired by this belief and connected to the elements, I fully believe the heart and soul are connected. As the heart expands, the soul brightens, and vice versa. When the heart builds a wall around itself, the soul becomes solid plaster and seals the cracks. The heart and soul balance each other and work in relationship to support us through the struggles and challenges of life. When we work on healing the heart, the soul will align and return to place of equanimity.

In chapter 2 I mentioned using a blue gemstone as a way to support healing. I often recommend crystals and gemstones to my students and gift them at retreats, and they have been part of my own toolbox for a really long time. Even as a little girl, I was always fascinated by the flicker in the my grandmothers' jewelry drawers. I would just sit, hold the jewels, and soak up the energy. Across the globe, crystals and gemstones have been part of ancient medicine and the transfer of energy through space and time.

For this next exercise, I invite you to use a moonstone in the meditation. The moonstone is a pearly, iridescent gem filled with powerful moon energy that can nourish and awaken feminine energy. As a healing guide, it leads you through the inner workings of the soul, washes away negativity, evokes sensual tranquility, and resets the mind and body. As a calming and balancing gem, it is connected to the crown, third eye, and heart chakras.

HEART & SOUL MEDITATION

Come into a comfortable seated position on the floor or in a chair. Place the moonstone in the palm of your right hand and place your right hand in the palm of your left hand. Close your eyes and breathe lightly in and out of your nose. Do this for fifteen to twenty breaths. As you breathe in, focus your attention on the center of your chest, the heart chakra. Feel the energy of love, compassion, forgiveness, and understanding flow through. Keeping your breath light and smooth, feel the energy radiating from the moonstone. If you aren't intuitively feeling it, don't worry. Simply focus on the breath and relax. Allow the gem to do the work. Remembering the colorful rays and glimmers of light in your stone, imagine N'Game pulling back her bow and directing healing arrows into the wall around your heart. As each arrow pierces the wall, your heart and soul feel lighter, open, and free. Do this for as long as it feels right for you.

At the end, press the moonstone into the middle of your chest. Inhale deeply, hold your breath for five seconds, then exhale slowly out of your mouth. Repeat two more times. Slowly open your eyes, and if you desire, feel free to journal.

PRESS REPLAY

As you've probably noticed throughout the book, journaling plays an essential role in releasing, shifting, and activating energy within the body and mind.

Way beyond writing down random thoughts and intentions, journaling is a great stress-management tool that lowers blood pressure, strengthens the immune system, and improves your memory and mood. But one of the major aspects is that it nourishes the emotional body, which in turn starts to punch through the weak blocks of the wall. We become more present with our feelings and self-confidence begins to shine through. As self-awareness deepens, so does personal growth. As the blocks begin to fall, we become more creative in the way we view, engage, and live in the world.

Gratitude journaling is a lovely way to drop into the heart, but I prefer acknowledging daily life experiences. As we see the beauty in each day, our heart begins to live more abundantly in the field of hope, and possibilities become realities. The most practical, spiritual, and self-nurturing exercise is a process I call Replay the Day. This nightly meditation and journaling exercise creates a space to visually see your heart moments mentally and on paper. Mostly, it gives you time to reflect and experience them again. By hitting replay in your mind, your heart and soul are able to feel and acknowledge the day's events. This reduces self-loathing thoughts by genuinely highlighting the positive or neutral states of being even within a challenging day.

REPLAY THE DAY MEDITATION & JOURNALING

Before you start, make sure you have your journal and pen next to you. • Come into a comfortable seated position on the floor or in a chair. Close your eyes and breathe softly in and out of your nose. • Take about fifteen to twenty soothing breaths. Once you feel calm, start to think about a single moment in your day that touched your heart. • As you visualize this moment, reconnect to the feelings you experienced within your heart without judgment. Do this for two to three minutes. • Then for another two to three minutes, release the replay button and be in the present moment.

At the end of the meditation, slowly open your eyes and write down the entire moment from your day in your journal. Include the tangible elements and the emotions you felt. Close the journal, close your eyes, and take three deep breaths in through the nose and out through the mouth. Repeat this exercise for the next fourteen days and observe the powerful shift in your life.

BURN DOWN THE WALLS

OMG! This heart thang ain't easy, and allowing yourself to feel the emotions of the heart makes it even more difficult. Somewhere between love and loss, prisons are built as mechanisms to shield ourselves from the pain. The fascinating part is that even though we have a deep desire for love, the wall continues to get higher and the maze leading to freedom becomes more complex. If we're willing to acknowledge our fears, unearth our own dysfunction, and create personal steps to change, anything is possible. As you know from my words and thousands of posts on Instagram, self-love is vital on our path to self-realization, but this work goes beyond saying, "I love myself." The real question is, "Do you love yourself enough to knock down the wall and set fire to that shit?" Are you ready to expand your heart and initiate a new way of living in spiritual freedom? Are you ready to love so passionately that your relationships on all levels become more vibrant and fulfilling? In order for this to occur, you have to commit to the hardest work of all. You have to commit to a forty-day practice.

The practice is forever guiding me on a journey called *growth*!

Within the practice of yoga, there's the word *tapas*. In Sanskrit, *tapas* comes from the root word *tap* meaning "to burn." Traditionally it is often linked to words like *austerity* and *discipline* and involves having the self-discipline to burn off impurities. As a tantric thinker, I believe we are all divine, and we are created with the oneness of God merged within our soul. From that perspective, I am not trying to burn the so-called wrong or bad aspects of myself. I am not trying to eliminate the shadows and little demons. Instead, I am working toward living, breathing, and loving *all* that I am. Within the practice of personal alignment, the goal is to create heat and inner friction in order to become the best version of yourself, which is God. It's easy to sit behind the glass walls of cloudy illusions and give the impression of rainbows, unicorns, and personal empowerment. But the deep work happens in the fire, heat, and brimstone. I'm not telling you to torture yourself or practice yoga twice a day, I'm inviting you to realign to your highest self through purification practices and daily rituals with the goal of burning away the pain and mental constructs you've placed around yourself.

Tapas is also connected to *svadhyaya* (self-study) and *ishvaraprandhana* (bowing or surrendering to a higher power). Like many of us steeped in a world of technology, it's easy to bypass these two concepts, but we also know that intimate

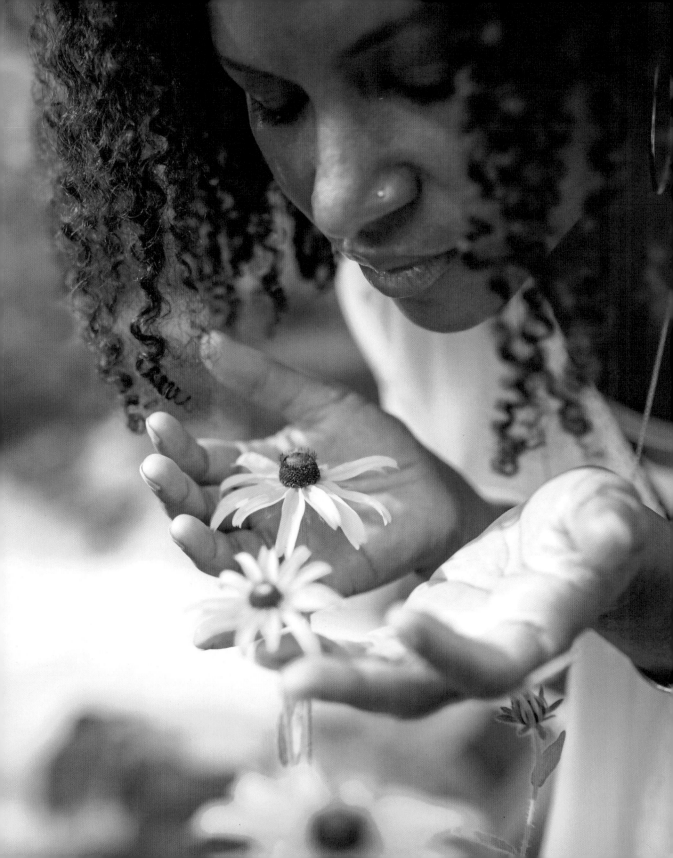

personal reflection and acknowledging a higher power requires connecting to uncomfortable sensations. So instead of hiding behind walls, following the norm, masking our feelings in addiction, projecting our fears onto others, and swimming in low vibrational experiences, we need to jump into the fire. We have to commit to engaging multiple tools and spiritual technologies to thoroughly decontaminate the mind, body, and soul.

FORTY DAYS OF DEVOTION

I'm constantly looking within the depths of my soul to find clarity, intimate connection, and the answers to the hardest decisions in life. But mostly, I'm looking within to enhance my relationship with the *soul,* and ultimately, God. My relationship with the energy or higher power I consider God has been the strangest of love affairs. I often think of it as a high school crush that turns into the best marriage after you've dated and divorced all the others twenty years later.

As a child, my inner vision of God was luscious and beautiful. The stories from pastors and biblical scriptures coated my heart with deep commitment and devotion. When the reality of HIV, death, and random disappointments shattered the vision, I was defeated. But upon finding yoga, God and I began dating as adults with baggage. I carried so much personal crap and built so many walls that I often ghosted God as well. Instead of facing the realities of life, I often avoided meditating (even though I knew it was good for me), and I purposefully ignored sacred messages within the exhales of my vinyasa practice. Like my tangible relationships, I would go strong for a few months and then dump God when the essence of my own divinity began to shine. Basically when I felt confident enough to speak from my heart or make bold choices for myself, I would crawl into my shell in hopes of not being seen.

Through a dedicated forty-day practice, I gained devotion from my heart and soul. I believe that my devotion elevates me. It builds a divine platform from which I can love, create, and evolve. If my spiritual foundation is soft and shaky, other aspects of my life will unravel and soon implode. But if my foundation is steady, I have the capacity to step into the best version of myself. As I've discussed, the majority of our pain and suffering comes from our habits. At the same time, our habits can cultivate joy, happiness, and peace.

Before we talk about why we are practicing for forty days, let me share the meaning of *sadhana*. In Sanskrit, *sadhana* is defined as a "process, discipline, or service that cultivates spiritual connection and inner peace." The act of discipline rooted in mindful intention and pure devotion enables you to surrender to the chaotic workings of the ego and opens a portal to the voice of God. Sadhanas are typically activities like meditating, practicing asanas, chanting, or engaging in morning prayer daily. For some, early morning practices work really well. My lifestyle and personality calls for a more fluid time for daily practice. As a Virgo, I'm all about the details and perfection. Giving myself a little freedom within a forty-day sadhana softens personal rigidity and enables me to commit to the practice without feeling like it's a chore. As I move, breathe, chant, and meditate, my daily sadhana generates love and devotion, uplifts my spirit, and heightens my connection to self.

rising and falling with
each breath
fire rushes into my soul
chanting along
the spine
as my pulse
silently races
tears maneuver
across the face
while my feet create
rhythmic circles
that awaken the spirits

A period of forty days is significant in a number of cultures and religions. In the Bible, a forty-day period is symbolically connected to a time of trials and spiritual testing. The most well-known one is Moses, who spent forty days and forty nights on Mount Sinai. But mostly, forty days is viewed as the length of time for transition. Within the practice of kundalini yoga, doing a kriya or meditation for forty days breaks negative habits that may be blocking us from personal expansion. My forty-day Heart and Soul on Fire sadhana is about shifting your connection to the self, unraveling years of dysfunction, and building a solid foundation. This energy-centered approach also kickstarts a new mindset and breathes positivity into your life. Organically, it enhances your relationships and enables you to reexamine the self-defeating patterns you hold in your heart. As you create a solid foundation, you naturally identify negative patterns and work toward refining your heart. Just for a few seconds, pause and review the assortment of relationships in your life. Notice how your state of mind impacts your relationships in a positive or negative manner.

During my first forty-day personal practice, I experienced the bliss of God return to my heart, and that sealed the deal. I knew it would forever be a major tool for burning down the walls. Here's how it could potentially go. Somewhere around Day 6 or 7, you may want to quit. If you don't quit, by Day 14 you may feel the emotional toxins gush through your pores. Literally, you smell differently. As Day 21 rolls in, you will intuitively know you are on the right path, and as things feel more comfortable in the practice, other aspects in your life start to shift organically, often in ways you least expect. By Day 30, you may fully and authentically feel God within you. It's almost as if the universe starts to dance with your soul, and your heart is returning home. By Day 40, the practice is medicine.

yoga & meditation practice
forty-day heart & soul on fire sadhana

After consistently engaging in other practices throughout the book, you are more than ready to dive soul-first into a deeper experience. As you move in the practice, I recommend getting clear about why you are traveling on this spiritual path. Knowing your motivation and intention will greatly support you on those days when intense feelings and toxic emotions bubble up. Let go of the heady projections and focus on your feelings, aspirations, and heart-centered desires.

mantra

Ong Namo Guru Dev Namo.

When crafting your intention for the Heart and Soul on Fire sadhana, follow these simple points: (1) write in the present tense, (2) be specific, (3) use affirming and positive words; never state what you don't want, (4) believe it in your heart, and (5) use words that generate a feeling and deep emotion each time you read them. Once you have written your intention down, place it somewhere you can see it every day.

INTENTION   Read your intention out loud. At the end, place your left palm over the heart chakra, and the right palm on top of the left hand. Breathe slowly in and out of your nose for at least one minute, feeling the beat of your heart and soaking in your intention.

SUFI GRINDS   This is definitely one of the ways I like to get the fire stirring. Along with releasing tension, this flowing movement directs energy upward from the base of the spine to the crown of the head. It massages the internal organs and aids in digestion, and when it's engaged with deep breathing, it's a great way to cleanse and renew the internal system. When you close your eyes, you drop in to a soulful vortex similar to the spinning motion of the devotional dance of the Sufis.

HOW TO PRACTICE   Come into a seated position and cross your legs. Place your palms face down on your knees. Close your eyes, and on the inhale, move your upper body to the right, forward, and to the left. On the exhale, draw the spine back and to the right. You are creating a circle with the upper body. The movement should be smooth and continuous and effortlessly flow with the breath. Do this for one minute, then reverse the direction. Return to center, take a deep inhale, hold the breath for three to five seconds, then exhale. Be still for another five to ten breaths and observe the sensations within the body and mind.

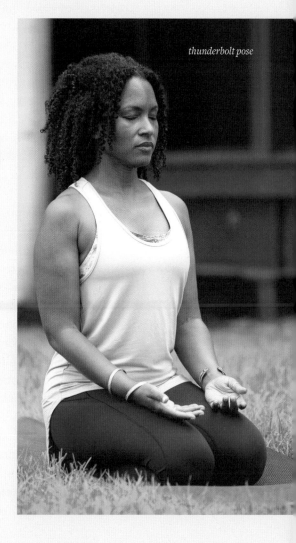

thunderbolt pose

THUNDERBOLT POSE (*VAJRASANA*) WITH BREATH OF FIRE   As a posture that's often used in meditation, Thunderbolt Pose strengthens the back muscles and core and fine-tunes spinal alignment and posture. The elongation of the spine lengthens the front of the body, opens the chest, relaxes the shoulders, and enables the breath to travel freely.

Breath of Fire is rapid, rhythmic, and continuous with equal-length inhales and exhales (on average two to three cycles per second) through the nose. The power is generated from the navel and solar plexus, and you should expel the air out by drawing the navel toward the spine. Pairing Breath of Fire with the Thunderbolt Pose amplifies the engagement of the core, which increases digestion and purification. In addition, more clarity is gained because there's a clear and open pathway of energy moving upward toward the third eye and crown of the head.

HOW TO PRACTICE   If you have sensitive knees or ankles, grab a blanket or towel to support you in the modifications. Kneel on the floor and sit on your heels with your feet relaxed. If this is uncomfortable for your knees, place the blanket between your calves and hamstrings. Another option for your knees is to sit on the blanket and allow your feet to rest outside the blanket. Use as many blankets you need to sit with ease. For discomfort around your ankles, slide the blanket under the tops of your feet and ankles. If none of these work for you, come into a cross-legged position. Place your hands on your thighs with the palms facing up. Keep your shoulders relaxed and your spine straight. Close your eyes and practice Breath of Fire for one to three minutes. At the end, breathe in and hold the breath for five to ten seconds. Then exhale with force through the mouth. Repeat this two times.

Caution: Do not practice Breath of Fire if you are pregnant or on the first few days of your moon cycle.

CORPSE POSE (*SAVASANA*)   Probably one of the most difficult postures to fully experience, Savasana is about releasing, surrendering, and allowing the body and mind to let go. It calms the mind, relieves stress, and is the ultimate total body relaxation. I often tell my students to "allow the earth hold you." Often reserved for the end of a yoga class, this posture can be done anytime you need it. Use it as a way to lower your blood pressure and deal with insomnia, fatigue, and headaches. It can be done on the floor, on the sofa, and yes, in bed for a mini nap.

HOW TO PRACTICE   Have a seat on the floor, bend your knees, and slowly recline onto your back. Lift your pelvis off the floor, extend your tailbone toward your heels, and slowly lower your pelvis back to the floor. This action will help to lengthen your lower back and create ease. Straighten your legs and take your feet wider than hip distance apart. Relax your arms down beside you a few inches away from your body with your palms facing up and your fingers relaxed. If this position is uncomfortable for your neck, place a blanket or towel under your head. I also recommend placing a blanket or pillow under your knees to ease any tension in the lower back. Move and adjust as much as you need to. This posture is about full relaxation, so make it a sweet gift to yourself after the

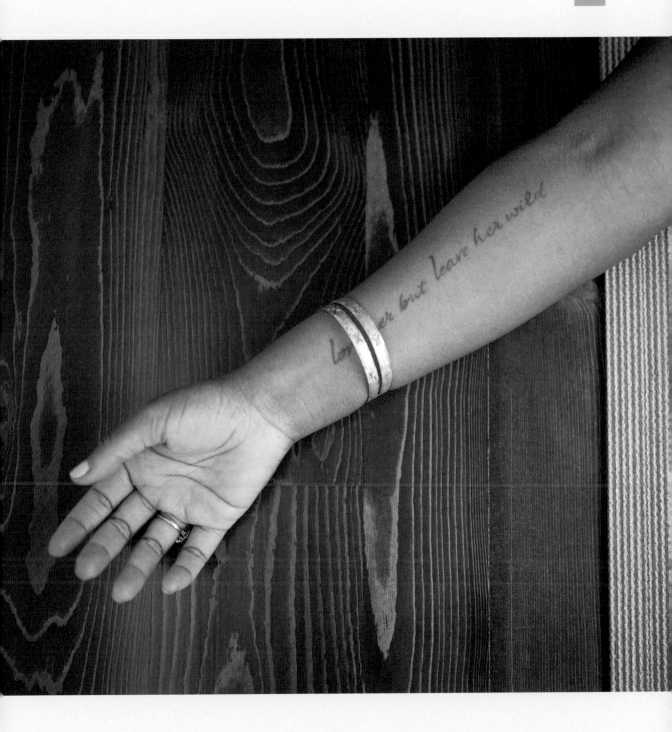

Breath of Fire. Take seven long, deep breaths through the nose. On each exhale, imagine yourself melting deeper into the arms of Mother Earth. Then release your focus on your breathing and just be still for three to seven minutes.

KUNDALINI MEDITATION: CALLING ON THE SPIRIT OF MOTHER EARTH

From birth, the soul penetrates the human and seeks to live out a path fueled with brilliance. Between the time of our birth and the present moment, we allow our souls to be pulled, twisted, and darkened. As you drop into this meditation, call on Mother Earth, call on N'Game, call on the fire within your soul to elevate your infinite power to be you.

HOW TO PRACTICE   Sit in a comfortable seated position with your legs crossed or sit in a chair. Create a soft neck lock by lifting your chest while lengthening the back of your neck and lightly pulling your chin toward the back of your neck. Relax your face and close your eyes. Lift your arms up into a 60-degree angle with your palms facing in, your fingers straight and together, and your thumbs relaxed. Visualize a flame at the center of your heart chakra. Hold the position and breathe long and deep through the nose for three minutes. At the end of the three minutes, inhale deeply and hold the breath for fifteen seconds, drawing upon the strength of Mother Earth. Then exhale. Repeat the inhale deeply again, and hold for another fifteen seconds. Feel the blessings of Mother Earth pour through your heart center. Exhale slowly. Repeat the cycle a third time, feeling a sense of love swirl around you. Relax your arms and rest your hands on the knees.

To close, open your eyes and seal the practice by repeating your Heart and Soul on Fire intention. Bring your palms together and inhale and exhale with an extended *Sat Nam*.

GETTING THROUGH YOUR FORTY-DAY PRACTICE

I know every day is not the same, and I've designed this practice to support just about any lifestyle. Give yourself about twenty to thirty minutes for the full practice. This gives you time to chant, read your intention twice, move through the asanas, and drift into the meditation. If you don't have enough time for the full practice, split it into two parts. In the morning, practice the opening chant, intention, asanas, and the closing mantra of *Sat Nam*. After work, complete your day with the opening chant, intention, Call on the Spirit of Mother Earth meditation, and closing mantra of *Sat Nam*. The key is not to work yourself up or feel overwhelmed if you don't have time. By the way, this practice also works if you are traveling. If you keep a copy of your intention on your phone, it can be done anywhere, even in the airport.

The sadhana is crafted to reset your natural rhythm as it extracts and detoxifies old patterns embedded in the body, mind, and soul. Energetically you will feel uneasy at times, and certain days will be more difficult than others. Be with the sensations, give yourself time to feel what's bubbling to the top, and breathe through the uncomfortable with love and compassion. Know that you are digging below surface emotions, and these forty days are about creating space for the soul to be renewed.

Love in all its forms rests within each beat of the heart. As we breathe, cry, and feel the pulsation of experiences, our soul absorbs the sensations and pushes this energy into every inch of our being. It doesn't matter if the sensations are glorious or deathly uncomfortable, the subconscious mind records the message. This recording is replayed when we are triggered, and it repeats over and over when we are in the depths of sadness. Regardless of the event, the heart feels and the soul remembers. So in the split second of pain and trauma, we begin to build protective walls around the strongest yet most vulnerable pieces of who we are. The more pain the heart feels, the higher and more layered the walls become. Then we arrive at a place where the heart is surrounded by a maze of sadness. In a state of shielding ourselves, emotional detachment becomes the heart's autopilot and our current state of living. We stop experiencing the fullest of divinity and internal expressiveness of our spiritual form.

In the darkest hours, light always seems to shine through. It may come in the form of a memory, a friend, or even a random stranger who demonstrates an act of love "just because." This simply means there's a crack in the wall, and where there's a crack, there's hope. Within the tiny cracks of light, the subconscious pushes forward memories of possibilities. In the glow of possibility, we are able to see and know it's going to be okay. We begin to see the potential of something different. We begin to realize sadness and pain don't control who we are. Crack by crack, we learn the tools of coping with pain and how important it is to move compassionately through the darkness and simmering emotions.

As more light penetrates the heart, the sovereignty of the soul begins to rise. Beautifully connected as cosmic dance partners, the heart and soul nurture us crafty humans through relationships, struggle, hardships, and uncertainty. It doesn't matter the tools we select during the process, our natural state of being is full expansion and freedom nestled in the heart. The cracking of the wall through meditation, breathwork, and even journaling serves as an intentional step toward balance. Where the soul breathes, the heart glows; where the heart opens, the soul flows.

With the wall still present and only bits of light touching the heart, it's really easy to fall back into old patterns. Especially if the universe drops a painful bomb you've never experienced. Sadness and despair find comfort in the pain, and you attempt to seal the cracks. However, that's the time you have to ignite a fire. It's actually the universe telling you to wake up and turn your patterns into rubbish. Through a committed and intentional forty-day practice devoted to purifying and opening heart-centered energy, the love resting within you becomes your normal. Therefore, by knocking down a few weak walls and setting a fire to the entire fortress, you are blazing a new path for your heart and soul to glow.

dancing circles around the sweetness of my soul
folding into rose tainted waves of emotions
leaping through a lifetime of dreams
remembering the sound of sensual bliss
distant echoes fall upon my face
lilies covering my path of hopes
as the morning twists my belly into a shy
the taste of fire clearing the way
my heart ripples to the top
I recall the feeling of openness

trust & have faith in yourself & others

*a*ll the walls are white, but I see darkness. I keep gazing, and wondering when I will feel liberated from emotional discomfort. I've done the work, chanted the mantras, and sat in stillness for hours. But I'm only feeling the smallest of shifts. My physical body is strong, and I'm not triggered as much by my pain. I definitely feel more rooted in myself, confident in my abilities, but for some strange reason I don't have the capacity to trust people. I constantly second guess their words and wonder if their actions are pure. As I stare into nothing, I begin to ponder. Do I trust myself? Is the doubt I have with others simply a reflection of my own thoughts? After days of soul searching, I realized that I'm also incapable of making the hard decisions for myself. Somewhere along the path, I stopped trusting some aspect of my own power. I stopped trusting the woman I know I am.

For some reason in the Spring of 2013, the topic of trust was on my mind. Throughout my life, I've made my own decisions and confidently moved into action with full commitment. But in the moment and stillness, I uncovered the reality that I needed to unload another layer of fear and breathe fiercely into life choices. Although I had spent the last year and a half working through my emotional pain, I still wasn't free. I was doing the work, burning down the walls, and feeling *a greater sense of love within, but something was still missing. I had lost FAITH in myself and everyone around me. That's when I decided to retool the gauge of trust in order to fully be Spiritually Fly!*

At birth, we have no choice but to rely on the acts and deeds of others. Within those relationships there's an element of blind trust that guides our connection, love, and adoration for adults. As time moves on, we experience betrayal in the form of words (spoken or unspoken), physical violation, or emotional infringement. While we are learning the experiential lessons around trust, we are also learning insecurity and doubt. As children we learn to wear the mask of shame around being ourselves, especially if we were told "children should be seen and not heard." The fascinating part is, this statement was originally used in reference to young women in fifteenth-century English culture. Within religious forums, it was okay for women to be present, but they were not allowed to contribute to the conversations of men due to their so-called innocence and naivety. Since this phrase has been so commonly used generation after generation, it's no wonder that as adults we have major self-trust issues. Not only is there a trust imbalance with others, but there's also a major struggle within ourselves.

Along the vast landscape of spiritual teachings and religious institutions, we are also taught to believe and have faith in the unseen. One of the definitions of faith is the "strong belief in God or in the doctrines of a religion based on spiritual apprehension rather than proof." As I've shared, my faith in God was unwavering in my youth. I fully believed in the power of prayer, and my proof was a perception acquired from my mother and grandparents. But the moment my brothers were diagnosed with HIV, I felt myself drifting further and further from a belief in all things. My view of life drastically shifted when I discovered meditation and yoga. Even after I began practicing, I was more likely to put my trust in an arbitrary God on a cross than look within for the answers. Not until late 2012 did I truly find myself sliding into alignment with the magical moments of the God within.

I'm sure you are thinking by this point in the book that you have this life mastered. NOT! Life is forever evolving. The steps on the spiritual path of uncertainty can sometimes guide us to issues we thought were resolved. So yes, there's more work to be done. Now is the time to strengthen your trust muscle and to breathe love into faith.

DECODING RELIGION

I have a feeling that what I'm about to share will rub people the wrong way, but I've learned it is important for me to share my true journey. Over the years, as my relationship with God was renewed, the following biblical scripture continued to surface. The passage was one I would hear on any given Sunday from Baptist pulpits, and I vividly remember it during funerals and family memorials. I recall the day my dad was being buried. Between the men carrying his body to the grave and cries during the twenty-one-gun salute, the pastor read this scripture. The first line is what I couldn't seem to work through. I struggled for so many years with the religious aspect of God, and I watched in anger as my mother suffered in silence over her life's experiences. How can we trust a God that doesn't believe in humans? How could we, over and over, give our hearts to a God that hasn't comforted us at our lowest points? How could we possibly lean in with an open heart, when horrific occurrences in life pollute the strength we have in spiritual teachings and humanity?

> Trust in the lord with all your heart and lean not on your own understanding; in all your ways submit to him, and he will make your paths straight.
>
> PROVERBS 3: 5–6

When the internal dialogue around trust surfaced in my mind, I knew I had to evaluate my personal interpretation and understanding of the Bible. Basically, the lack of belief based on my own meaning of God was weighing on my heart. That heaviness thrust me into hours and days of reading, meditating, crying, and listening to gospel music. I laugh now, but I know my yoga students knew something internal was happening. I would play old church hymns as background music during classes and give dharma talks about knowing the self. When things got really confusing, I would read blogs on religious topics in hopes of finding an answer or something to provide comfort. It was a spiritual puzzle I was committed to piecing together, and by the grace of God I was determined to find clarity.

Months and multiple forty-day practices later, I finally found comfort in knowing that trust and faith are key elements of spiritual teaching regardless of your religious beliefs or not. As simple as it may sound, our ability to commit to a forty-day practice is trust and belief in the self. Even my ability to share openly about my personal struggles around religion with friends and students was an act of spiritual bravery. But mostly, having the capacity to rethink valuable life teachings and retool them for modern life took enormous personal growth. This concept and inner dialogue enabled me to expand my heart beyond my childhood imagination. It also set the final stage for one my biggest challenges in life . . . trust and faith.

My Interpretation of Proverbs 3: 5–6

It only makes sense that Proverbs 3: 5–6 is one of the most quoted passages in the Bible. It touches on so many elements that we mere mortals deal with daily. Life experiences and personal choices send us on what sometimes feels like the most unforgiving ride. The heart opens and contracts, and at some point the muscle becomes fatigued and stops moving. By sharing my interpretation of this passage below, it's my hope that the Bible and other religious texts can be used as nurturing sources of spiritual growth regardless of your beliefs.

> Trust in the lord with all your heart
> (*Trust your inner voice that is the heart and soul*)
> lean not on your own understanding
> (*when making decisions, don't allow the mind to rule*)
> in all your ways submit to him
> (*surrender to the heart*)
> he will make your paths straight
> (*when you listen to the heart and soul, all will become clear*).

In the Arms of Faith

Faith is alive in all phases of life. It starts the moment we take our first breath, it waits patiently as we question our existence, and it welcomes us home when all else fails. We feel faith when the words "I love you" pull us off the ledge of panic and fill us with joy in the bliss of celebration. Faith never judges, never condemns, and never refuses access. Too often we get lost in the stories of not believing, and we leave faith on the side for the religious fanatics. In reality, faith is all there is, all that will be, and faith will forever open her arms to receive you with grace.

I breathe with gratitude, trust, and faith while my heavenly guides illuminate my path.

As I guide you further through my real-life interpretation of Proverbs 3:5–6 below, you will realize faith is a matter of connecting to what's inside. Faith is the endless source of divinity living within you. It's just a matter of recognizing it as we make decisions on a daily basis.

Trust your inner voice that is the heart and soul. The concept of pausing to listen is part of all spiritual teachings. From meditation to prayer, it is essential to create space so the inner voice has somewhere to speak. Our busy lives are masterpieces of chaos and in order to trust the inner voice, time must be allocated to be. By now you've experienced different types of meditations, but what about when you don't have time to be still? That's when you begin to cultivate "mini mindfulness moments" in your life. These are moments when you thread breath and quiet time through normal daily activities. For example, walking your dog, taking a shower, folding clothes, and even washing dishes. I'm always amazed when divine thought rushes in while I'm walking my dog Sebastian. As you breathe in a state of conscious awareness, the mind, heart, and soul make space for intuition

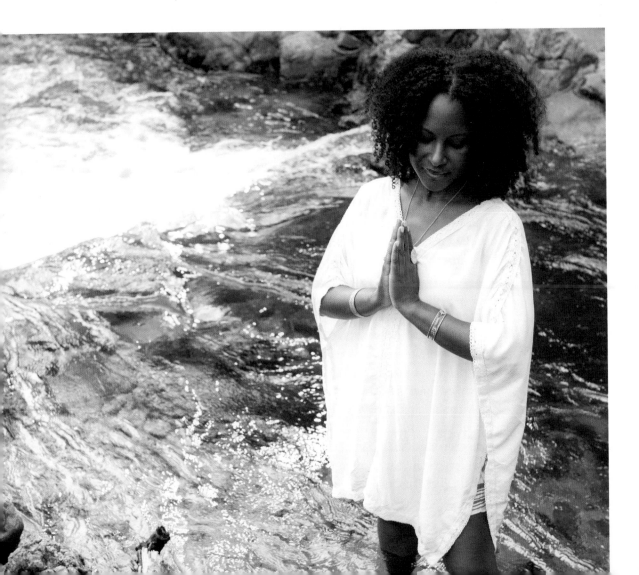

to come forward, and we simply know without knowing how we know. We know from a place of internal awareness and intuitive personal connection.

When making decisions, don't allow the mind to rule. As the inner voice comes through, give yourself the flexibility of knowing the inner voice may appear in the form of a feeling or emotional sensation. As feelings drift to the source, they're trying to get your attention to go right, left, or down the middle. You may label them as "red flags" in bad situations, or they may come through as bodily roars such as goosebumps when a decision feels right. As much as our minds are powered by thoughts, faith is powered by an inner knowing.

Surrender to the heart. Within the American work culture, we are guided heavily by the mind. This starts in school when we are instructed to memorize and logically process information. Children are rarely asked how they are feeling or encouraged to make decisions based on feelings. As the body feels, the mind steps in with a big chop. The mind-over-heart state prevents us from listening and following what we know is the truth in our hearts. When your mind attempts to take control of your heart, I recommend taking a few deep breaths and circling back to the option that appeared initially. When you return to your first choice, you release fighting the mind, and surrender to the heart.

When you listen to the heart and soul, all will become clear. Big decisions are complicated and often impact the lives of others. That means the mind pushes, tugs, and battles the heart on a higher level. It places the heart in a state of confusion and emotional pressure and masks the feelings with fear and anxiety. In this situation, you have to exercise compassion and give yourself time to pull apart the pieces of emotion and internal anarchy. This includes creating an expanded space for listening, recognizing the various types of emotions moving through you, and truly sitting with your heart's desire. I describe it as having a "soul talk" with yourself. Weighing all the options, moving along the path that's most aligned with your truth, and telling yourself that regardless of the outcome, everything will be okay because you followed your inner voice.

Following this approach with simple decisions is always a good place to start. Try it when you're deciding which way to drive to work or what you should plan for meals that week. As faith builds, move into larger, more complex decisions. A beautiful meditation that I often recommend clients practice when their decisions are filled with confusion is the Grace of God meditation.

KUNDALINI MEDITATION: GRACE OF GOD

This glorious meditation is designed to evoke and manifest grace, strength, and inner radiance. It channels positive energy, strengthens the weak spots within the soul, increases clarity, and enhances communication. As it balances all five elements within our being, it merges our limited ego with divine will. It is one the best meditations when our faith is being tested by outside forces, when a hard decision needs to be made, and within those periods when our inner god or goddess isn't communicating with the heart. This meditation enables us to rise into our divine fullness.

HOW TO PRACTICE   Rest on your back with your eyes closed and your entire body relaxed. Inhale deeply, and as you hold the breath, repeat silently ten times, *I am the grace of God.* Tense the fingers one at a time to maintain the count, then exhale completely. Before inhaling again, hold the exhale out and repeat the mantra ten times again. Repeat this for a total of five inhales and five exhales. Ultimately you will silently repeat the mantra one hundred times. • When you have completed the five full mantra breaths, slowly sit up into a cross-legged position with your eyes closed. Place your right hand in gyan mudra (see page 45) with the back of your hand resting on your knee. Lift your left hand to shoulder height with the palm facing forward. Breathe at a relaxed and normal pace. Starting with the little finger of the left hand, bring tension into one finger at a time and repeat the mantra five times for each finger on both hands. At the end, simply relax and meditate for a few more minutes.

SEEDS OF SELF-TRUST

Within the self-help and wellness industry, the phrase "be yourself" has become a power mantra. From yoga teachers to life coaches, there's massive emphasis on expressing and living as "yourself." I've realized that having the capacity to live fully in this world as oneself requires courage, strength, and a constant act of patience. Personal growth and development don't happen overnight, as you've experienced in your forty-day practice; it takes time and compassion. In the constant quest of refining myself, I determined that trust and faith impact my ability to "be myself." Over the past eighteen years or so, I've realized that tiny seeds were planted, and it was up to me to water them, trim the weeds, and revel in their beauty as they grew and I got older. The seeds planted by my parents and other adult figures of my childhood grew, but periodically life would cut the flower before it bloomed. There were also moments when my soil would become contaminated with fear, insecurity, and doubt. Self-worth, self-awareness, and self-confidence are three major seeds that support your ability to trust and have faith in yourself. By default, when this occurs, you have the confidence to trust and have faith in others.

Self-Worth

To know your worth is to know your value, and we touched on this in chapter 3. But I wanted to also share that self-worth is wrapped in the cradle of self-esteem. In the current world of social media, it is so easy to base your self-worth on external factors such as imagery, comments, or cultural behavior. My father was excellent at reminding us of our worth, but not until adulthood did I realize how many self-worth seeds were planted within childhood lessons. One lesson of self-worth happened one day after gymnastics class. The look of defeat was all over my face, and at the age of seven, I knew my gymnastics dreams would soon come to an end. While leaving the gym, my father asked if I wanted to play on the swing. Like any kid, I said yes. As we walked over he asked if I enjoyed gymnastics. Not understanding what he was building up to, I responded yes. He followed up with a few more questions around my likes and dislikes and by the time we made it to the swings, my father had determined that my favorite aspects of gymnastics were the warm-ups, floor exercises, and balance beam. The movements came natural to me, and I caught on to them with ease. The uneven bars and the vault were not my jam, and I was always embarrassed to do them. On that day I had face-planted into the vault, and even my strongest Virgo willpower couldn't pull me out. Somewhere in between the questions and a few pushes on the swing, my dad dropped a seed of self-worth into my little being. By emphasizing what I was good at and stressing that my determination to be the best was an admirable quality, my dad magically uplifted my spirit and reminded me of my worth. On top of that, as a girl and a woman of color, he constantly emphasized that my color did not define or dictate my path. As I share this short story, I can hear him loud and clear: "Don't forget to psych yourself up! You are ready! Do your best because you are great!"

SELF-WORTH ASSESSMENT & JOURNALING

Close your eyes, take ten to twenty breaths, and return to your childhood (somewhere between the ages of one and thirteen). See if you can locate a situation or person that planted a seed of self-worth within your soul. Visualize the full experience—what brought you to that moment—and recap how you felt. After about three to five minutes, open your eyes and write down everything you can remember from your visualization. Then write how this self-worth seed has grown and impacted your adult life. If by chance you didn't have water and fertilizer for this seed, don't worry. Write how you can take this memory and replant it in your current life.

Self-Awareness

It is easy to coast through and just allow life to happen by mentally drifting, settling for the ordinary, and allowing others to guide and control our lives. Self-awareness is about having a deep inner knowledge and understanding of our character, strengths, weaknesses, feelings, and desires. Philosophers from various cultures have all agreed that one of the biggest challenges of being a human is to "know thyself." As powerful beings, having self-awareness is a seed that grants us the super strength of conscious acts rather than passive occurrences. It is also a seed of wisdom to be brave enough to see, accept, and rely on your gifts and talents to support your own evolution. It can be a difficult process to uncover the inner workings of who we are, but even more challenging to face and accept our strengths and weaknesses. As a trainer, I'm always ecstatic to watch trainees awaken to a new strength or magical gift. In yoga teacher training it happens around the time they begin designing their own sequences based on the techniques and theory. This glorious moment happens because other trainers and I have encouraged and guided trainees down the path to confidence with reassurance and support. From the beginning, we identify something unique within them. With a nurturing word or glance, we highlight their strengths and supportively share their weaknesses. In this learning environment, trainees see themselves more clearly and are blown away by their new ability. In the end, they become much more aware and the burst of confidence fertilizes their soil.

SELF-AWARENESS CHECK-IN

Call three friends, coworkers, or family members. Make sure the individuals you select can be super honest and forthright. Tell them you are working on refining your level of self-awareness, and you need them to share three strengths and three weaknesses about you. These can be general overall observations, or they can be connected to your job, family, or how you treat yourself. Make sure they understand that you are creating a safe and open-hearted dialogue. What they share will be held in a place of love, and you will be receiving it as a tool to become a better person. In addition, what happens during this conversation stays in the moment. It should never be discussed unless one of you asks to do so in another safe environment agreed upon by each of you.

After the conversation, sit silently and breathe for two to five minutes. I just want you to feel everything. If you become anxious or start to cry, it's okay. Breathe slowly and feel the feels. At the end of your meditation, journal about the entire process. Write about what was shared and what you felt in the moment and then answer the following questions for each strength and weakness.

STRENGTH

How are you utilizing this strength in your current life? Is there room for improvement?

WEAKNESS

How is this weakness holding you back from being the best version of yourself? Does this weakness match up with or relate to a shadow? If so, how can you work emotionally with this weakness to become more self-aware in daily life?

Self-Confidence

As we water and fertilize self-worth and awareness by believing in our abilities through trial and error, personal evaluation, and maintaining that belief through the challenges, confidence begins to organically grow. Receiving reassuring comments and praise is great, but it still takes extra effort to blossom into your full potential. I believe one of the major steps to self-confidence is taking control of your life. That means taking solid, grounded actions that enhance and improve who you are and how you live in the world. So far, all of the steps you've taken have been major action steps, but they have mostly included a lot of releasing and unearthing of old habits. My teachings are definitely rooted in positive affirmations, but I also wanted to bring up the reality that sometimes negative thoughts will pop into our minds. Within the wellness community, many teachers will tell you that pushing the negative thoughts away will keep them from impacting your level of self-confidence. I'm here to tell you that it will not. Let the negative shit bubble to the top, feel it, acknowledge it, and know it's simply a little demon knocking at the door. From the seeds of self-worth and self-awareness, self-confidence will rise covered in Golden Glitter.

SEEDS OF CONFIDENCE MEDITATION & JOURNALING

What if you didn't have someone in childhood helping you to positively shape your thoughts, or if during adulthood a traumatic experience poisoned your healthy stems? How do you reach your goal of being fully worthy and confident? Don't worry; after all this shedding, you have the capacity to lift yourself up. This meditation is a beautiful positive-affirmation approach to individualized growth.

Come into a comfortable seated position on the floor or in a chair. Close your eyes and begin to breathe deeply through your mouth. Take at least five to ten breaths. Seal your lips and allow the breath to flow naturally through the nose. Start to visualize the highest version of yourself. In your mind, begin to see yourself engaging in acts of personal strength. See and feel the strengths your friends and family shared during the check-in. Also feel strengths you know about yourself. Imagine yourself navigating life with ease, fully absorbed in your strengths. Do this visualization for three to five minutes.

At the end of the meditation, describe the following in your journal:

* The highest version of yourself you saw during your meditation
* What makes you unique
* Your best character traits
* A moment in your life where you felt the most powerful
* Three words that you would like to live by
* How you surprised yourself this month

Now close your eyes, sit in stillness, and breathe slowly for another one to three minutes. Slowly open your eyes and begin to read out loud the following affirming statements. Repeat the affirmations over and over for one to two minutes. Feel free to create and add your own affirmations.

* I am happy and joyful.
* I am kind and compassionate to myself.

- I love the person I am now and am becoming.
- I am competent, smart, and creative.

As the seeds of confidence begin to grow, something magical starts to happen. You feel free to "be yourself," and you know without a doubt that you have the power to make your own life choices.

IT'S IN THE GUT

We've all heard or used the phrase "trust your gut." It's that feeling or reaction we experience in the belly described as intuition. Our intuition has a beautiful way of tickling the belly, whispering in our ears, and guiding us on a path based on our deepest feeling. But when there's a lack of personal trust, we ignore the sensations and fail to listen to our highest guru . . . the Self! I can't begin to tell you how many times I've heard my inner voice talking and thought I was just being paranoid. One of those instances was when I opened my first yoga studio in DC. I remember sitting in the building owner's office going through the lease, and my "gut" was telling me something wasn't right about the space and the business partnership. I ignored the sensations and moved forward because I really wanted to open a studio. Within a year, I had numerous disagreements with the building owner, the studio was robbed three times, and I was teaching six days a week while also working a full-time job. Within two years, we moved to a new location, but honestly the studio never soared. By the end, my business partner and I disagreed about everything, and I didn't trust her. In full disclosure, I didn't trust myself, and I didn't believe in my own skills as an entrepreneur.

Our third chakra (Manipura) rests in the region of the body above the navel and the bottom of the rib cage, and it harnesses our self-confidence, self-esteem, and ability to make decisions. When this realm is out of balance, we may suffer from digestive issues, eating disorders, poor body image, insecurity, the lack of drive, and yes, fear of rejection. Often called the fire of material consciousness, the third chakra has the capacity to detoxify the body and mind. On a physical level, it impacts the kidneys, liver, gallbladder, spleen, small intestines, stomach, diaphragm, and the solar plexus. Through the process of unraveling trust in 2013 and my work with women, I determined that it is essential to do daily third-chakra practices in order to build confidence and maintain the work that has been done. It doesn't matter if I'm teaching a vinyasa/flow or kundalini practice, tapping and purifying the gut must be done. I find the single most effective practice is Stretch Pose.

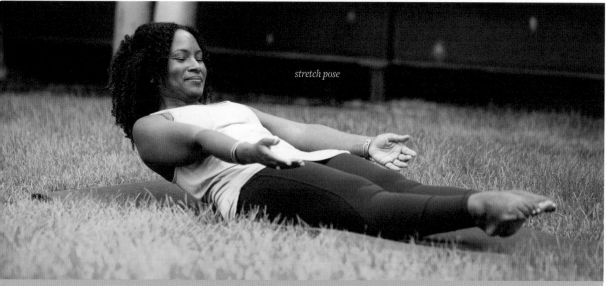

stretch pose

STRETCH POSE

This pose blends Breath of Fire with an intensive physical posture. It fires up confidence, supports one's efforts to release fear and insecurity, purifies the blood, strengthens the abdomen, and resets the entire nervous system.

HOW TO PRACTICE   Recline on your back and extend your legs with the toes pointed and legs together. Press into your lower back while lifting your head and heels six inches off the floor. I recommend lifting the head and shoulders before lifting the legs. Extend your arms straight over your legs with fingers straight and palms facing down but not touching the legs. Hold the posture and do Breath of Fire for one to three minutes. If you have lower-back issues, place your hands under your buttocks. Don't stress if you can't keep both legs off the floor. You can lift one leg at time while doing the pose but remember to keep the legs and arms straight. At the end of the designated time, inhale, hold the breath and the posture for five seconds, then exhale and relax the body and breath.

IN TIME WE BUILD

While working on cultivating self-trust, I find it rewarding to expand my faith and build trusting, loving, and mutually supportive relationships. There are many methods and techniques for building these relationships, but the most valuable resource is time. Regardless of whether you're cultivating a relationship with a romantic partner, a friend or coworker, or a family member, don't rush in. Pace yourself and move with kindness, not fear. This is a gradual process that involves feeling safe, confident, and secure around this person (emotionally and physically). You have to be the judge on the amount of time it takes. With an open heart, rooted in truth, and layered with keen self-worth and awareness, you will know and have the willingness to trust and have faith in others.

As you navigate and build this mutual commitment of trust, I recommend you consider the following actions for cultivating trust in a relationship as part of your personal process of spiritual growth:

- Communicate. Start off with zero ambiguity. Let the person know you are working toward building trust and a strong relationship. Within that, clarify your expectations around a healthy relationship, always make time to listen, never be afraid to share, and ask questions when there's uncertainty. Clear and concise communication is the foundation of all relationships.

- Be authentic. Lead from your highest realm of self-worth and self-awareness. Always show up as your truest self, and never hide who you are. Don't compromise who you are just to get closer to someone. Trust me, when they see and feel the real you, they will embrace all of you.

- Lead by example. If you want someone to trust and have faith in you, you have to model the behavior you expect. Within that, stand firm, and offer what you desire. Never do or give more than your capacity.

- Be your very best self. Show up with kindness, love, and understanding; people tend to fall in line and want to be better as well.

- Evaluate periodically. Relationships are fulfilling for both parties. Trust can't grow if only one person is open and willing.

Know it is important and totally okay to evaluate the
relationship to determine if it's working for both of you.

- Be dependable. Do what you say you're going to do and
  approach the relationship with integrity. Demonstrate qualities
  of reliability, take responsibility for your own mistakes, and
  know it takes courage to speak your truth and apologize.

- Be open. It's okay to share your deepest thoughts and feelings
  and the qualities that make you beautifully human. At the same
  time, be respectful of the other person's vulnerability.

- Be supportive. We all need someone to lean on. Say and demonstrate how
  much you care and be of service without expecting anything in return. Be
  a cheerleader with honesty and be generous with your compliments.

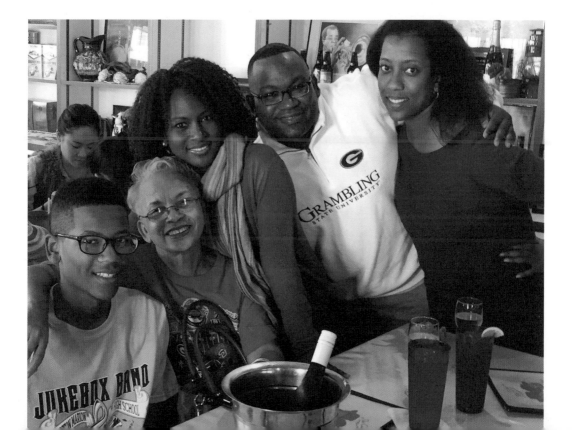

yoga practice
cultivate trust & faith

One of the best ways to cultivate trust and faith is by feeling and experiencing it in the body. Active movement pushes us on a physical level, but it also test us on an emotional level. When you think you can't go any further, the breath engulfs the tangible and carries us beyond our comfort zone. There's a beautiful element of trust that moves past the mind and breathes effortlessly into the heart. In a matter of seconds, the arms of faith extend a cradle of reassurance.

mantra
I trust and have faith
in my divine wisdom.

LOW CRESCENT POSE (*ANJANEYASANA*) Low Crescent Pose stretches and strengthens the groin, hip flexors, and quads. With the lift of the chest and arms, it opens the front of the body, stretches the lateral sides, and also improves core strength. Energetically it is a very open and expansive posture for the heart.

HOW TO PRACTICE Come into a low lunge with your left foot forward and slowly lower your right knee to the floor. If you have sensitive knees, place a blanket or towel beneath the knee. Relax the top of the right foot on the floor if that's comfortable. Take a deep inhale, and on the exhale move the hips gently forward to deepen the stretch along the quad and groin. Be mindful not to push the left knee too far past the left ankle. On the inhale, slowly lift your arms overhead while keeping your shoulders relaxed. Your palms can touch or you can keep them slightly apart (shoulder distance). As you hold the posture and breathe for five

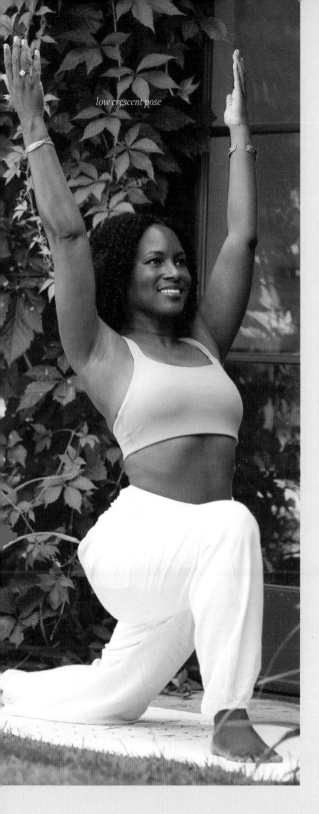

low crescent pose

breaths, isometrically draw the left hip forward and the right hip back. Extend the spine, lift the sternum, and reach the fingers toward the sky. As a modification, you can always rest the hands on the front thigh. Repeat on the opposite side.

MONKEY/SPLIT POSE (HANUMANASANA) This posture can sometimes create an enormous amount of fear in individuals that have tight hamstrings. On an energetic level, this is not just about easing tightness in the body; the posture also teaches us to trust and have faith in ourselves through the devotion of planting seeds of spiritual growth. It strengthens the abdominal and pelvic muscles, stretches the hip flexors, increases flexibility and the range of motion of the legs, and improves overall alignment through the engagement of the lower body.

HOW TO PRACTICE   If your legs are super tight, I definitely recommend doing a few gentle leg stretches before you do the posture. From the Low Crescent Pose, place both hands on the floor next to the front foot. Breathe in, and on the exhale

REVERSE TABLE TOP/ALTAR POSE

(ARDHA PURVOTTANASANA)

This pose drops you immediately into the energy of trust because as it stretches the shoulders, chest, abdomen, and spine, the entire front of the body is elevated and exposed and the head is released. This openness is invigorating and energizing and helps with fatigue and emotional stress. It's also a complete physical offering of letting go. Along with stretching, it builds strength in the core, arms, wrist, and legs.

HOW TO PRACTICE   Have a seat on the floor with your legs extended. Bend your knees and place both feet on the floor hip-bone distance apart. Reach your arms behind your hips shoulder-width apart. Slowly lift the pelvis while pressing the palms and feet firming into the earth. Make sure the weight is evenly distributed. Hold for five deep breaths. Repeat three times.

reverse table top/altar pose

gently draw the hips back as you straighten the front leg (don't lower the hips toward the back heel). This position is called the Half Split Pose and may be a good place to stop if your legs are too tight to go deeper. To continue, slowly slide the front heel forward. If the front heel is sticking, use a towel or blanket under the heel. As you extend and move into the full expression, isometrically draw the front and back hip toward each other. This will help to keep the hips stabilized and the pelvis level rather than overreaching through the legs. Keep your spine straight, the crown of your head lifted, and your shoulders relaxed. Use blocks under your hands as support if you can't move fully in the posture. Hold for five breaths, then repeat on the other side.

CLOSING MANTRA Find a comfortable seated position. Place your right palm over your belly and your left palm over your heart center. Close your eyes and chant the mantra *Ram* seven times to seal the practice.

KUNDALINI MEDITATION FOR *BROSA* (TRUST)

As I've discussed, trust and faith start within. Once you settle into a place of ease, then you can begin to expand your reach to others. This meditation directly affects trust emotionally and energetically.

    HOW TO PRACTICE Tune in by chanting *Ong Namo Guru Dev Namo* three times. Sit comfortably in an easy crossed-legged position or in a chair. Lift your arms over your head in an arc (elbows slightly bent). For feminine energy, place your left palm over the top of your right hand. For masculine energy, place your right palm over your left hand. Place the tips of your thumbs together with the thumbs facing back. Gaze softly down toward your upper lip.

    Hold the posture and chant in a light whisper *Wahe Guru* for three to eleven minutes. *Wahe Guru* is "Wow . . . Oh my God!" It represents the indescribable bliss of going from darkness to light.

    Close the meditation with a long *Sat Nam.*

From cultural imbalance, based on outdated norms to adult inadequacies, we struggle constantly with knowing, trusting, and having faith in what we think and feel. Even though the modern interpretations of spiritual texts are outdated, we are still more inclined to believe what a minister or "holy man" says is truth than to trust our own knowing and divine inner voice. We have failed over many lifetimes to read the texts and form a relationship with God. However, this practice is about unearthing the norm and creating shifts by connecting to the God within. Through self-study and questioning, you are able to see behind the surface and grow flowers of belief.

By reevaluting the words and God and placing my hands to my heart, I was able to plug into what made soulful sense to me. It all came down to plowing my own fields, planting seeds, and honoring what's within. That means you have to make time, even during mundane tasks, to start listening. You have to acknowledge the roars and goosebumps, then be okay with the decisions you make. But in reality, you have to have an intense soul talk with yourself and believe the answers are within.

No matter how we are moving through life, it all comes back to the "self." It's impossible to have a lasting romance or a great career if we aren't constantly breathing into the concepts of self-worth, self-awareness, and self-confidence. These are the three prime seeds for growing the foundations of trust and faith. To know your worth is to know your value. Self-awareness is about celebrating your strengths and being unafraid to face your weaknesses. And through self-worth and self-awareness, self-confidence has the liberty to root and expand.

As fire blazes in the belly and penetrates the heart, belief in yourself is restored. With restored belief comes waves of intuitive life choices coated with the Golden Glitter of trust and faith.

bask in your unforgettable brilliance
twirl along the lines of magnificence
drop petals in the waters of creation
sing lullabies to your future as the
mother cradles your soul

SUTRA 6

follow your passions with conviction & purpose

i t was late 2013 and Lizandra Vidal, a DC yoga teacher who was living in Haiti post-earthquake, reached out to me and inquired if I was interested in supporting her efforts in the country. As you can imagine, my response was simply, "Yes!" My yes went beyond the American desire to do "good work." The mission behind her efforts drew me in because of my Louisiana roots, eclectic bloodline, and my "sista love" connection to all women. As women, the breaths of our souls are carbon copies of each other, and there's nothing I wouldn't do to support women-driven programs. Regardless of the languages we speak and our countries of origin, as women we feel each other, heart to heart, soul to soul. Our lives may be different, but we are all at risk of abuse, rape, and violence.

On my first ride into the chaotic downtown of Port-au-Prince, I knew from the pulse of the city I was home. I always feel a powerful sensation upon returning to my place of birth, Louisiana.

Oddly enough, the same comfort trickled into my soul as I watched cars, mototaxis, and hundreds of people move about in their daily routine. My eyes periodically locked with several beings, and somehow our spirits merged in a wave of cosmic oneness. This was the start of my passionate love affair with Haiti. My trip wasn't a "mission vacation," but rather the continuous expression of passion in action. It is my dharma, my ultimate purpose in life, to be present, feel, and give from my heart. This trip was an opportunity to connect with the women and children of this beautiful country on common ground. Although there are challenges and a mix of daily struggles in a country of mountains, I opted to drop into a place of just being. "Island time" became my friend, and Haiti became my lover.

As in many countries around the world, including the US, women in Haiti are largely underserved and make up a large portion of the at-risk population. Inspired by Lizandra's commitment to empower girls and women, I knew this was the place I needed to be at this time in my life. Both Lizandra and I understood the principle that when we invest in girls and women, the whole community benefits. Thousands of international and non-governmental organizations had worked in Haiti since the earthquake, but many of them had only focused on stabilizing the country's infrastructure. Lizandra's efforts, Project Zen Empowerment and Ayiti Yoga Outreach, went beyond providing basic services. Her projects were rooted in giving people the option to experience peace of mind within the chaos. Through the practice of yoga and meditation, the inner self is fertilized and the outer self is stabilized to handle the struggles of day-to-day Haitian life.

You may be wondering why I fell in love with Haiti. The only answer I can give is that when I am there, I feel grounded. Like Louisiana, there's a warm vibration infused in the people, music, and culture that heats the soul. I feel plugged in to the source of spirit and wrapped affectionately in a blanket of resilience. Regardless of the fight, Haitians seem to have a resourceful way of responding and recovering, which is a fundamental quality many of us have lost in the modern world, especially the US. We are consumed by gadgets, express our feelings through texts, and experience life in an instant. We rarely view ourselves as spiritual beings, give respect to our ancestors, or make time to heal and connect purely with others. As a result, we are helpless when a real crisis challenges our coping skills.

During the first trip, my yoga was about breathing heart-to-heart with the people. Within my first forty-eight hours, I taught yoga to Haitian women and expats, played and practiced with a delightful group of school children who once resided

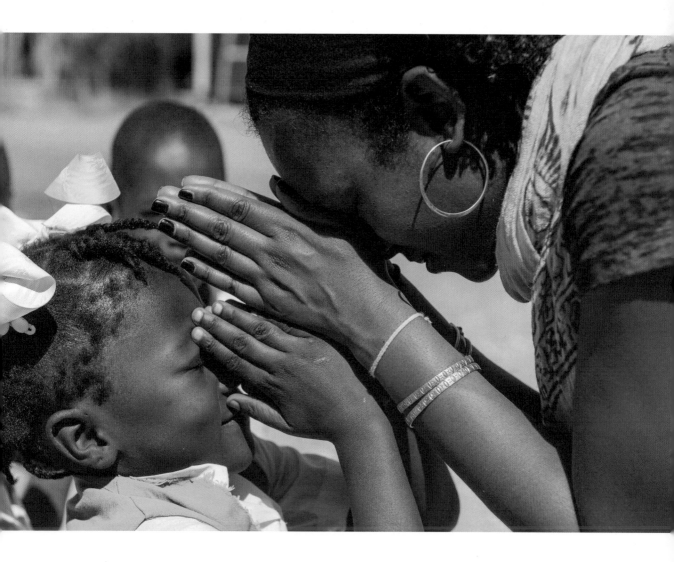

in tent cities, delivered yoga mats to girls in an afterschool program operated by the YWCA, and hiked downhill to visit a family of nine who lived in a two-room shack. These hours of extreme emotion and spiritual discomfort pulled on my heart in the way you yearn for your lover to return home. One special moment happened when my palms came together to acknowledge the divinity in a group of school children. The instant I said, "Namaste," they ran over with excitement to acknowledge the divinity in me. To this day, I've never experienced such a powerful seal of love. As you can imagine, I soaked in every single moment with an open heart filled with gratitude and passion. By the third day, I found myself drifting into a place of comfort and softened into a simple state of knowing. I was right where I belonged . . . I was in the arms of my lover . . . Haiti!

Months later, I returned to cohost a service/culture/yoga retreat. The retreat was open to all who desired to share and mentor a dynamic group of young adults on their journey of becoming yoga teachers. Unlike typical yoga retreats, I wasn't doing it to make money. I simply wanted to share what I loved most about Haiti and spend time training future teachers who lived in some of the toughest and most underserved neighborhoods of Port-au-Prince. The second visit magnified my soul and reinvigorated my passion as a yoga teacher. During my first visit, by inspiring the women of Haiti to nurture themselves and change their communities via the practice of yoga, I supported Lizandra's vision to empower young adults to create change within themselves and their community. But this time around, Haiti empowered me to look at ways I could reshape my work and create more avenues to serve the needs of women around the world. Since that time, I have magnified my passion, expanding and creating more programs and opportunities for women of all races and backgrounds to learn, grow, and heal together. Although this book can be used by all, you can probably tell that I had women on my heart during the development process.

PASSIONATE COSMIC DREAMS

Within the threads of the story above, you may have noticed the sweet layers of conviction, purpose, and love. It doesn't matter if you are associating passion with work, a cause, or even a deep desire within you, passion is the strong wave of emotion that inspires you to live from the heart of your being. Passion whispers tender reminders in your ear, sends creative pulsations through your veins, and keeps you energized for days. Without a doubt, passion feels and often occupies your mind like a never-ending romance with the greatest lover. In reality, it can be hard to drop everything, move to Bali, and make jewelry on the beach. However, you were born with a well-spring of gifts, talents, and passionate cosmic dreams. As a natural by-product of purifying the soul, there will automatically be a surge of passion moving to the surface.

I say this with a firm voice: It is your right and responsibility to fulfill your passionate dreams. You may think it's unrealistic or unattainable, but you at least have to try. Not trying will leave you frustrated, angry, and resentful. If you recall working with your demons, you may notice how one of the shadows is associated with a dream or passion not followed. Often the passionate dreams we had from ages five through twenty-five were suppressed or crushed as a result of shame, pain, or adult controls over who we should be. At some point around our Saturn return, the passionate dream starts to surface. It may appear in the same form as a childhood fantasy or emerge looking completely different while holding the same cosmic energy.

Before I continue, I should probably explain what a Saturn return is. It is when the planet Saturn slowly and beautifully loops back around to meet your natal Saturn. Every twenty-seven to twenty-nine years it orbits around the Sun and returns to the same sign in which you were born. You start to feel the pull in your late twenties, and it continues to impact your life into your thirties. A second return happens around ages fifty-seven to sixty. This cosmic ritual is a spiritual alarm. It blasts you into major shifts, requires you to access your current state of being, and with loving force teaches some of the biggest lessons. Saturn is the teacher, and during the return it teaches you to overcome while showing you patience, stability, reliability, and diligence. But here's the crucial piece: Saturn will buzz everyone's chart, but not everyone will wake up and do the work. In most cases, people will assume they are experiencing a rough patch, or that life just sucks, or from childhood programming, that this is just how their life is designed. As a result, they never seem to wake up, or when they do, it happens with such a drastic shift everyone around them is in shock.

Living out our passions before, during, and in the middle of our Saturn return is about reconnecting to our dreams and intimate longings. We do this by connecting to our inner child. That joyful, playful, blissful dreamer creating in the ether of fantasy. One of my clients was having a difficult time at work and was passed over multiple times for promotions in her communications firm. After a few chats, I realized she had lost her creative juice. Along with working on her second chakra and doing some shadow work, I also encouraged her to visualize her most creative memories of childhood. To her surprise, she had created a toy theater, always colored outside the lines, and enjoyed dancing. I recommended she do one of the following: volunteer at a local theater in any capacity that excited her, paint weekly, and go dancing as much as she could. She opted for the latter two, and within a few months she was promoted to a new position. As a bonus, her intimate relationship with her partner improved as well. Communication and creativity were her gifts and passions, but in the midst of daily life she lost the starry-eyed child. She lost the dreamer who crafted playful story lines and comfortably colored outside the lines. By returning to the memories and incorporating the energy of her inner child, my client was able to bring forth the energy of dreams into her current reality.

DREAMWORLD MEDITATION & JOURNALING

This meditation should take about five to ten minutes (stay and dream as long as you wish). Grab a towel or eye pillow to block out all the light. Use your favorite 852 Hz Solfeggio frequency recording. Tuning into this frequency helps us awaken intuition and return to spiritual order. I find that when we are tapping into the source of our inner child, we are returning to a place where earthly inhibitions don't exist. It is the space filled with celestial energy and extraterrestrial imagination.

HOW TO PRACTICE Turn on your music and come onto your back (use a pillow under your knees for support). Cover your eyes and make yourself comfortable. Take ten to twenty slow breaths through your nose. Relax your body starting with the soles of your feet and moving up to your face. Guide yourself slowly through each part of the body and allow the breath to assist you in the process. Once you feel at ease, visualize your hand reaching out to open a door. On the other side of the door is a room filled with all your favorite toys, colors, and images that make you happy. It may include items you didn't have as a child, and that's okay. This is your dreamworld, so fill it with whatever items you wish. Now begin to see yourself playing and doing the things you enjoyed as a child. Do what brings you joy, makes you laugh, and creates a feeling of bliss. Stay in this place and enjoy. When you are ready to come out, take a deep breath in your dreamworld, open the door, and slowly return to the present moment. Take five deep breaths in through your nose and out through your mouth. Gently rise and take out your journal.

JOURNALING

Write what you most remember from your meditation. List what you felt, what you played with, and the things you did.

OBSERVATION

What energy or aspect of your dreamworld can you thread into your current life?

THE PASSION OF KARMA AND DHARMA

Since I graduated from college, a common thread of service has been woven throughout my adulthood. It is heavily stitched into the colorful fabric of all I do. In assessing the lives of my parents, I found that their common thread was also service. My father was in the army for twenty-plus years, and my mother was a teacher and an employee of the Department of Human Services in Louisiana for over twenty years. Today she's an elected official in the state of Louisiana. So as you can see, serving my community is definitely something I know well. But this is bigger than following in my parents' service footprints; my service is my dharma, my purpose. Service is my *Passionate Purpose*!

This brings me to the epic text called the Bhagavad Gita, often referred to as "The Song of God" or "The Song of the Lord." The Gita is a story within the Mahabharata, and it is a poetic dialogue between Krishna and Prince Arjuna of the Pandavas. Arjuna is on the battlefield and gazes across to see his family and friends, the Kauravas. He throws down his bow in chapter 1 and refuses to fight because of an internal struggle and moral dilemma around good, evil, and human life. He seeks guidance from his charioteer, Krishna, who imparts the wisdom of pure devotion and selfless action. Within the seven hundred verses, Krishna responds to the prince by constantly urging him to fulfill his duty and fight. This is the core: karma and dharma.

Dharma has been defined as "duty, order, or law," but mostly "path of action or righteousness." *Karma* is defined as "action" or "work." As they play upon each other in the Gita, it is Arjuna's dharma, his path as a warrior, to engage in war. His duty must be fulfilled so he may live in highest consciousness; therefore, in order for Arjuna to complete his cycle of karma, he must fight. In the end, he fulfills his dharma and fights the battle.

Within our modern framework, I view dharma as the path of action that fuels the soul. If we are traveling along the road of our true purpose and committed to the process from the heart, the beauty of life will unfold. I'm not saying it comes without a struggle, but I do believe your soul is at peace when you step fully into your dharma.

I witnessed dharma in action through my older brother, Michael. At a very young age he wanted to become a doctor, and everything prior to his death focused on that path. In the early years of the AIDS epidemic, the medications used taxed the body and caused various side effects. Michael's cocktail caused dizziness and nausea, and this impacted his ability to effectively practice medicine, so although

> O Arjuna, when one performs his prescribed duty only because it ought to be done, and renounces all material association and all attachment to the fruit, his renunciation is said to be in the mode of goodness.
>
> **BHAGAVAD GITA 18.9**

he knew that not taking his medication would lower his T-cell level, it was more important for him to serve and live out his dharma as a doctor. Although his death caused me a tremendous amount pain and sadness, I finally absorbed the concept of dharma when I felt the fullness of my purpose. I understood his drive as the sparks of purpose flared in my being. Tingling, butterflies, and goosebumps appeared on a regular basis. The mystical messages were clear, and I was finally listening with the divine willingness to fulfill.

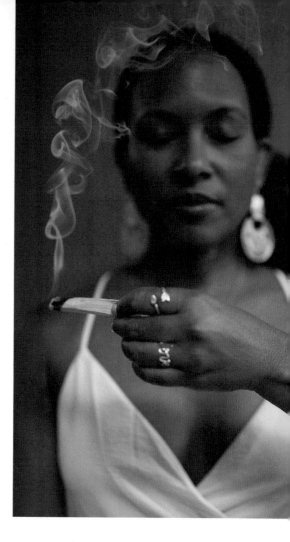

I know what you are thinking: teaching yoga and meditation are my dharma. No! These practices are tools I use to enhance my personal and spiritual life, and they are the tools I share to live out my dharma. But my true dharma is *to be of service by empowering and inspiring others to live their lives as divine beings.* An expression of my dharma is to help people live a Spiritually Fly life! By knowing your grand purpose, it is easy to see and follow the things you are passionate about. Basically, it was easy for me to say yes to Haiti, and it is fun to uncover new projects that always seem to circle back to my dharma.

WHAT IS YOUR PASSIONATE PURPOSE?

If you feel lost and confused on your path, don't freak out. It can sometimes take years to uncover your dharma. It did for me, and I'm sure it did for millions of others around the world. Within the trappings and confines of social norms and parental directives, we are blinded to what's deep inside. Hopefully by now, the practices in this book have supported your efforts in peeling back a few layers and tapping into the gifts that rest within. I also hope these practices have cracked

PASSIONATE PURPOSE EXERCISE, PART 1: CREATING

We rarely make time to dream big or think about what truly makes us unbelievably happy. Therefore, I need you to make this a major event. Give yourself about an hour or more to go through this exercise. Grab a cup of tea, light candles, burn palo santo, or whatever makes you feel at ease. The most important part is to find a quiet place where you won't be interrupted. If you wish, select a special journal and call it your Passionate Purpose Journal.

All the answers may not come to you the first time around. Don't force the process. The first attempt is usually about stirring your thoughts and stimulating your glorious insides. In the journal, reserve one section for your lists and answers to the questions and another section for those aha moments you will surely have. Up to this point we've been digging and purging, but now it is time to spray Golden Glitter everywhere.

STEP 1: MEDITATE AND LIST YOUR LIFE

Find a comfortable seat on the floor or in your favorite chair. Close your eyes and take ten to fifteen deep breaths to get out of your head and into your heart. Sit in stillness for another minute and just be. Then open your eyes and list the following:

- Ten to twenty activities that bring you joy and make you happy
- The common threads that run through those activities

- Personal strengths and skills you perform with ease
- Your successes and failures throughout your whole life (Write these without judgment and make sure you list the successes first)
- What you learned from your failures that gave you the strength and courage to move forward

STEP 2: MEDITATE AND CREATE YOUR PASSIONATE PURPOSE STATEMENT

Make yourself comfortable again. Sit or rest on your back. Place both palms over your heart center (left palm over the center of the chest and right palm over the left hand). Focus on your breath. Don't force or control the breath, just observe your natural breathing pattern. Also notice the beat of your heart for the first few minutes. After about two minutes, shift your thoughts to the activities that bring your joy. Visualize yourself fully engaged in these activities and notice the feelings associated with them. After five or ten minutes, let go of those thoughts. Simply be in stillness with your breath; feel and notice what surfaces to the front of your mind.

When you come out of the meditation, journal for one minute. Write whatever comes up for you. Then from your heart, create a statement that fully reflects your Passionate Purpose. Sometimes it helps to just write appropriate words down first and then come back to the full creation later.

you open and made space for you to see there is a path that is "your own." Passion and purpose move along the same lines, and the next exercise is designed to help you refine your Passionate Purpose. You've done a great job at calming the mind and releasing your fears, but now I want you to trust yourself and dream big. I want you to push overthinking aside and realize that your purpose is in your soul. It has been sitting there waiting for you to wake up and take action. It tugs at your heart on the exhale, and calls your name in a crowded room.

LIVING YOUR PASSIONS

Now that you've identified the things that excite you, you're either confused or freaked out. I know it can seem a little daunting, especially if your mind is saying, "You have a million passions, and barely time for even one of them." The Passionate Purpose process takes time to work through on paper and feel in your soul. It's totally common for insecurities to arise and indecision to step in, and everyone procrastinates in the sea of change. You've come this far, and now is the moment to elevate. I want you to think back to the commitment and strength it took to work through your most challenging shadow. There was doubt, anxiety, missed meditations, and possibly multiple do-overs. The same tenacity and personal devotion is what will lift you higher and propel you into the life your desire and deserve.

I am always amazed at how the lives of my yoga teacher trainees shift after they graduate. I've seen everything from marriage, divorce, and breakdowns to new jobs, quit jobs, and major relocations. Part of this has to do with what I call the "luminosity effect." This means when you hang out, absorb, and bask in the radiant, electromagnetic Golden Glitter of someone else, it pierces your soul. You see the qualities they possess, and you start to see yourself in them. You begin to realize that all is possible, and where your current seat in life is no longer okay. Your dreams become bigger, your hopes are seen as achievable, and your passions become more purposeful. It's not that you want to become these people, but that there's something about them you admire.

Within a group of trainees from all walks of life, there are many personalities and hundreds of life decisions. As they share, connect, and learn from each other, they also have the opportunity to absorb my glitter and the glitter of other trainers. Within the glorious mix of it all, the trainees are not only coming out with new skills and expanded gifts, but they've also experienced a massive wave of the luminosity effect.

Identifying your passion is only the beginning. Actually breathing it into existence requires a brave heart and deep commitment to yourself. As you visualize your desire, you have to take tangible action steps to bring it forward.

STEP 3: MEDITATE AND GET CREATIVE

Find a comfortable seat on the floor or in your favorite chair. Close your eyes and take ten to fifteen deep breaths to get out of your head and into your heart. Sit in stillness for another minute and just be. Then open your eyes and make lists of the following:

- People you know or admire from afar that are living out some form of the statement you created. Your list may include people you know personally or indirectly through friends or family, and it can also include celebrities or people you only see online. Don't get wrapped up in their whole life. Just list their name and the aspect of their life that matches your statement.

- Ways you could potentially live out your statement through passionate activities or a career. These may include activities within your current job, a part-time or volunteer position, or an activity you consider a hobby. Don't hold back or overthink the process. Have fun and GO BIG!

STEP 4: CREATE A PASSIONATE PURPOSE ACTION PLAN

Select the top three ways to live out your statement through passionate activities or a career from the list you made above. Make sure these top three really light you up, because they are the ones you will work on for the next six months to a year. During this time you will also be setting short-term and long-term goals, practicing daily and weekly rituals, and performing weekly and monthly check-ins on your progress as described below:

- SHORT-TERM GOALS These goals include anything you can achieve in the next one to eleven months. I describe them as the "see, feel, and taste" goals. Two great examples are training programs and a new job.

- DAILY AND WEEKLY RITUALS (AKA ACTION STEPS) These are all the tasks, conversations, classes, self-care activities, meetup groups, money, and people resources you need to achieve your short-term goals. Be clear, set dates, and don't be afraid to ask people for help. This may also include connecting with people so you can experience the luminosity effect.

- LONG-TERM GOALS These are goals you wish to achieve within the next twelve months or more. Within this time frame priorities may adjust, or a short-term goal may shift and impact a long-term goal. An example of a long-term goal is going back to school for a degree or specialized training. These types of goals take much longer and require the completion of short-term goals. Keep in mind: the unexpected always happens, so it's important to know it's okay to be fluid in this area. See the big picture and stay true your overall Passionate Purpose.

- **WEEKLY AND MONTHLY CHECK-INS** It's important to stay motivated and connected to your Passionate Purpose.

On a weekly basis, read through your rituals and action steps, check off tasks, add items, and make a pivot if necessary. Monthly, determine if you are on track with your short-term and long-term goals. Make adjustments where needed and don't forget to celebrate when you meet your goals.

You can use the chart below to create your Passionate Purpose action plan or recreate something similar in your journal.

PASSIONATE PURPOSE ACTION PLAN					
PASSIONATE PURPOSE STATEMENT:					
Passionate Activity or Career	Ways This Activity/Career Serves Your Soul & Others	Short-Term Goal(s) (One to Six Months)	Daily & Weekly Rituals	Long-Term Goal(s) (One to Three Years)	Weekly & Monthly Check-Ins

PASSION IS COMPASSION

In the last bullet in the exercise above, I asked you to determine how your passion serves others. As you move into the world pursuing your passions, it is so easy to get caught up in the self and egocentric desires. Although this book is all about tuning into the self and refining who you are, ultimately you do the inner work so you may shine your highest self, inside and out, on the rest of the world. After all, what good does it do to leave the world behind while you're walking a path that leads only to the self?

As you share with the world, it is essential to hold steady in your truth, have clear self-awareness, and know your divine purpose in life. As you explore your Passionate Purpose, examine how it will impact the lives of others, including your friends, family, and community. Ask yourself, "Will my passion, acts, and deeds elevate and inspire others and enhance the lives around me, or will they only benefit me?" Don't worry, not all passions require a global reach, but it sure feels good to the soul when they enrich the life of at least one person.

> Add a drop of human compassion to your purpose.

Here's another twist. It's okay to set short- and long-term goals attached to money. As you process that statement, know that having the financial flexibility to pursue a passion can directly impact the lives of others in a variety of ways. For example, it can create a more stable family environment because you are listening to your soul and not sitting in a place of resentment and fear. You may also have the ability to reach more people and touch more lives with a passion rooted in compassionate service. Therefore, if you were afraid to add money as a goal, go back and add it now.

Another important thing to consider is patience. As you set goals and commit to your daily rituals, be compassionate and patient with yourself and others. As humans, it's so easy to swim in the pond of expectations. We immediately feel a sense of satisfaction when our expectations are met and drown when timing is bad or the unexpected happens. When we are impatient, we are less compassionate. Always shoot for the stars, but breathe into light rays with patience. The beautiful part is that patience can sometimes open the door to new opportunities or inspire your creative juices. Give yourself the space and freedom to achieve your goals at a healthy and balanced pace.

yoga practice
follow your passions

With passion comes playfulness, freedom, bravery, and strength joyfully merged with compassion and purpose. Below I've included yoga postures that will help you experience all of these qualities—either when you are in them, or when you come out of them and feel the sensations moving through you. Give yourself a moment to warm up with some of the gentler chest-expanding postures in the previous chapters.

mantra

I breathe passion into my purpose.

GODDESS POSE (*UTKATA KONASANA*)   Evoking the strength of all the goddesses, this posture is grounding and elevating at the same time. As feminine energy pours into an open chest, this pose heats the entire body, increases circulation, stimulates digestion by strengthening the abdominal muscles, and activates the second chakra. As you sink deeper into Goddess Pose, you stretch the groin, hips, and inner thighs. While teaching the pose, I typically have my students hold it for longer than five breaths. This intensifies the strengthening of the quads and inner thighs.

HOW TO PRACTICE   From standing, step your feet wide and turn them both out to a 45-degree angle. Spread your toes wide and balance your weight between both feet. Take a deep inhale and on the exhale, bend your knees. If your knees extend past your ankles, widen your stance, but keep your knees moving toward your toes. Engage the abdominal muscles to ensure that the tailbone reaches toward the floor, while also honoring the natural curve of your back. Lift your chest, keeping your spine long and your chin parallel to the floor. Keep breathing and reach your arms out in line with the shoulders.

You can also reach your arms overhead and bring your hands together in a Kali mudra by interlacing your fingers, crossing your thumbs, and firmly pressing your palms together as you extend your index fingers upward. This is a powerful mudra of transformation that invokes the energy of the goddess Kali. It activates the upper chakras and helps break through negative thoughts and patterns, and it can be used to elevate and inspire you or give you a boost of confidence.

Release your shoulders and hold the posture for seven to ten breaths. Rest for five breaths and repeat two more times.

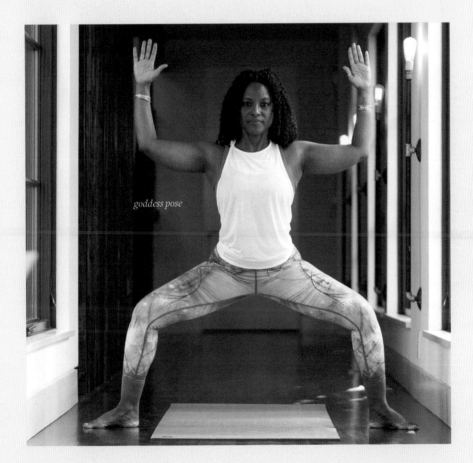

goddess pose

THREE-LEGGED DOG (EKA PADA ADHO MUKHA SVANASANA) A modified version of Downward-Facing Dog, Three-Legged Dog energizes and rejuvenates the nervous system, strengthens the arms and legs, stimulates digestion, and relieves headaches, fatigue, and insomnia. At the same time, it creates a yummy stretch along the hands, arches, calf muscles, and hamstrings. As energy flows through the hands to the feet, it dips into the hips and relieves stress and mild depression.

HOW TO PRACTICE   Come onto all fours, spread your fingers apart, curl your toes under, and slowly straighten your legs, lifting your hips up at an angle to where the ceiling meets the wall. Maintain straight arms and keep your neck relaxed while gazing between your legs or toward your navel. Think of creating a downward-shaped V with your body. Then, keeping both hands and your left foot connected to the floor, inhale and extend your right leg toward the ceiling, keeping it straight. There should be an inward rotation on both legs but especially the extended leg. It helps to think of drawing your big toe toward the

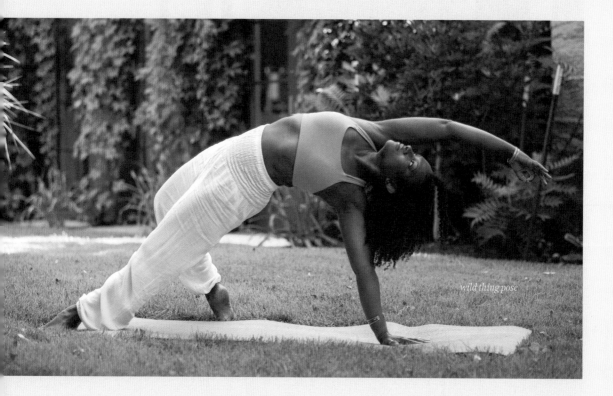

wild thing pose

center line of your body. This keeps your hips balanced. Keep your arms, legs, and abdominal muscles engaged. Hold for five breaths, then bring your right leg down, pause on all fours for a moment, then switch to the left leg.

WILD THING (*CAMATKARASANA*) The joy and playfulness of this pose spills over with cosmic exploration. It's grounding, yet free, open, and lighthearted. You flip into it from the Three-Legged Dog and throw it all to the wind with a big YES! It opens the chest, shoulders, lungs, hip flexors, quads, throat, and really the whole front of the body. The power of the posture cultivates strength in the hands, wrists, feet, legs, and upper back. It's also great for mild depression, fatigue, and insomnia.

HOW TO PRACTICE   From Three-Legged Dog with the right leg extended, shift your weight toward your left hand and left foot. With a slow transition, gently exhale, lowering your right foot toward the left side on the floor, keeping your right knee bent, your left arm strong, and your fingers spread apart. The right arm extends over the head while keeping the shoulder in its socket. As the ball of your right foot touches the floor, press your hips and chest toward the sky. Your right knee stays slightly bent, and your left leg is straight while you press firmly into the foot. Draw your shoulder blades toward each as your chest lifts higher. If it's comfortable on your neck, release your head gently back. Hold the posture for five breaths. To come out, I suggest lowering your hips to the floor. Repeat on the opposite side.

KUNDALINI PRACTICE: MAGNIFICENT NINE KRIYA & BEAMING PLUS CREATING THE FUTURE MEDITATION

With all the noise and pressure around us, it's easy to get distracted and lose track of our dreams, hopes, and deepest desires. Because you aren't the same every day, and the way we engage the breath and body can stimulate and soothe us in different ways, I've decided to share a full kundalini kriya and meditation in this section. It is a practice designed to boost your youth and inner beauty and improve your overall vitality (inner and outer), and on a physical level it massages the glands to release stress. I invite you to do this practice as a way to kick-start your purpose while you are exploring the potentials on your new journey. Like the yoga poses, it cultivates playfulness, freedom, bravery, and strength and merges them effortlessly with compassion and purpose.

The Magnificent Nine Kriya

The following kriya can be done as a stand-alone practice or just before another kriya or meditation.

HOW TO PRACTICE   Tune in by chanting *Ong Namo Guru Dev Namo* three times then move on to the following nine poses:

1. **CAT STRETCH**   Lie on your back and extend your arms out while keeping your shoulders on the ground. Bend one knee into the body and carry it to the opposite side toward the ground. Hold for a few breaths. Repeat on the other side.

2. **EYE OPENER**   Staying on your back, place your palms tightly over your closed eyes. Remain here and take a few deep breaths. Open your eyes and look directly into the palms of your hands. While looking into your palms, slowly lift your hands about eighteen inches above your face and continue to look into your palms for a few breaths. Place your fingertips on the center of your forehead and massage the area in a circular motion. Then gently move out to your temples, the sides of your face, and down toward your chin. Massage every part of your face including your nose, ears, and ear lobes.

3. **STRETCH POSE**   Remaining on your back, bring the inner arches of your feet together and point the toes. Press and flatten your lower back toward the floor. Extend your arms and fingers toward your toes with your palms over your thighs. Lift your head slightly, applying a neck lock by lifting your chest and sternum up while lengthening the back of your neck and pulling the chin back toward the neck, then gaze at the toes. Lift your feet six inches off the floor and do Breath of Fire for ten to fifteen seconds.

   Caution: Do not do Breath of Fire when you are pregnant or on the first few days of your moon cycle.

4. **COBRA POSE**   Roll over onto your stomach. Place your palms under your shoulders. Slowly lift your chest. Do your best to elongate your spine and relax your shoulders. Keeping your arms straight, begin to take long, deep breaths or do Breath of Fire for one minute.

5. **CAT-COW**   Come onto your hands and knees. Align your wrists and shoulders, spread your fingers wide, and align your knees with your hips. On the inhale, lift your chest and arch your back with your head and neck stretched up. Exhale and round the spine, drawing your chin toward your chest. Breathe powerfully and slowly; increase the speed as your spine gains more flexibility. Move constantly in the pose for three minutes.

6. **FRONT STRETCH**   Sit on the floor. Extend your legs forward and reach your hands toward your feet. If you can, grab your big toes with your index and middle fingers and thumbs (don't worry if you can't reach your toes). Inhale and lengthen your spine, then exhale and fold forward, with your chest toward your thighs and your nose toward your knees. Hold for several breaths. Avoid reaching with your head. You can also do this pose separately three times a day to check in and evaluate your mental strength.

7. **ROCK POSE**   Sit on your heels, placing your palms flat on your thighs. Do Breath of Fire for five minutes. An alternative is to sit on a block or pillow.

8. **FISH POSE**   Stay in Rock Pose and slowly release your torso back until your head and shoulders reach the ground. Hold for five to seven minutes.

9. **SHOULDER STAND**   Lie down on your back. Draw your knees toward your chest and place your hands on your upper hips. Extend your legs overhead and then lift them upward, so that your spine and legs are perpendicular to the ground. Your elbows and shoulders support the weight of your body, and your hands support your lower back. Without moving your head, press your chin into your chest and gaze toward your feet or close your eyes. Hold for five minutes.

Beaming and Creating the Future Meditation

Use this meditation as a way to project your future and your relationship with the world.

HOW TO PRACTICE   Come into a comfortable cross-legged position and sit with a straight spine. Place the backs of your hands on your knees in gyan mudra and close your eyes. Inhale a long, deep breath through a rounded mouth. Close the mouth and exhale slowly through the nose. Do this for seven to eleven minutes.

Next, keeping your hands in gyan mudra, inhale through your nose and hold the breath in. While you are holding the breath, if thoughts come to mind or emotions surface, "zero" them out. Exhale through your nose slowly when you need to, then repeat the breathing technique—inhale, hold, and exhale when needed—for seven to eleven minutes.

Finally, imagine a positive thought that reflects your overall desires and summarize it in one word like *health*, *knowledge*, *connection*, and so on. Focus on that single word and visualize its qualities. Inhale through your nose and hold the breath as you continuously beam and radiate the word. Exhale through the nose and relax when needed, then repeat the breathing technique—inhale, hold the breath, focus on your word, and exhale when needed. Do this for five to fifteen minutes.

Choosing a new path or taking steps into an area you've always dreamed about requires courage, emotional stability, an open mind, and the ability to listen to your heart. As much you may talk yourself out of something, remember it is your birthright to be happy. Part of that happiness is fulfilling your passionate dreams. It doesn't matter if you are twenty or sixty, your dreams are resting in your soul and waiting for you to set them free. Part of setting them free is tapping into your playful side, reconnecting to child-like joy, and remembering the fantasies we left behind in preschool. Once you do this, the fluid energy of the second chakra starts to move, and the soul starts to experience kisses of bliss with every smile on your face.

The path of action, duty, order, or cosmic law is your dharma. Like connecting to the celestial side of play, understanding your dharma aids in elevating the soul. There may be many paths on the journey, but when you set out guided by trust and faith, you have no other choice but to follow your dharma. Along the way you will explore your gifts, skills, and talents and at some point, a magical discovery appears in the form of a Passionate Purpose. There's no straight line, but by clearing and calming, you create the space to intuitively trust yourself and dream

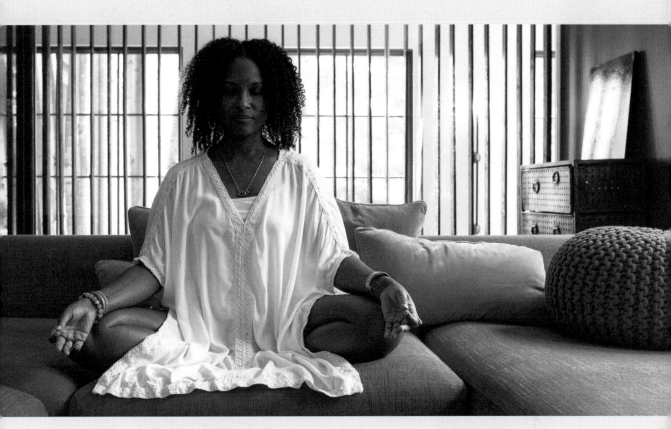

bigger than you ever have. Even in the random moments when fear attempts to tackle your dreams, you have the tools to see it and kick it to the side.

The hardest part of living is taking steps toward your Passionate Purpose, which requires you to shift from the dream state to reality. Doing this part of the work goes beyond daily affirmations and meditation. You need to write down your passion activities, set goals, and take daily/weekly rituals (action steps) to move into a purposeful life. These rituals serve as footprints on the path. They may include surrounding yourself with other amazing beings and experiencing the luminosity effect, committing to a daily self-care practice to keep your mind and body healthy, or asking friends to watch the kids one night a week so you can complete a few tasks. While it doesn't matter how you take the steps to live your passion, you have to craft a plan that keeps you focused and committed to your soul's purpose. Now that you have the tools, it's time to live your divine life without apology.

you are a mystical magical being
gracefully shifting
fearless in nature
taking brave steps into your future
breathing vast beauty into the universe
gliding across waves of uncertainty
cradled by your fierce heart
climbing mountains of change
while blowing gold dust
from your soul

SUTRA 7

be divine without apologizing

a s a young girl in Grambling, Louisiana, I dreamed of becoming someone great. From late nights in the dance studio practicing ballet to compromising my beliefs to make my lovers happy, my focus always centered on being perfect in hopes of gaining the praise of others. After years of peeling back the muck and reconnecting to my own heart, I finally realized it wasn't about becoming someone, it was all about elevating into my highest self.

We flow through life containing who we are and morphing into false images shaped by insecurity, doubt, and fear. Our external environment and what we call "life experiences" often dictate our beliefs and choices. Within the falsity of this existence, we drop into a level of normalcy. It's not until life gives us a really firm shake, do we stop, reevaluate, and opt to take a different approach. As I've shared, it can take years and continuous commitment to rise into our own sense of self. From my late twenties into my late thirties, God was calling and rattling my soul. Periodically I'd stop, listen, and shed a tiny layer of my own shit, but not until age forty did I fully peel back the layers and uncover my own divinity. At the point of surrendering, I determined it was my own divine inner light speaking my words of wisdom.

As you rise into your divine light, your soul can't help but lead you in a direction of living unapologetically. This doesn't mean crushing people in your path or refusing to consider the consequences of your actions. Living unapologetically means that you are living with openness, truth, purpose, and the deepest love of self. It means you are cultivating an intimate relationship with yourself and honoring every aspect of your being. Mostly it refers to being your *divine* self. Being that Golden Glittered goddess or god you see in your dreams.

I AIN'T SORRY

Why do I need to apologize for doing what makes me happy? Why does it matter if they judge me for my choices? Why do I have to say I'm sorry when sharing my feelings? These questions often surface when we are in the middle of navigating this new way of being ourselves. Living unapologetically can easily make us feel guilty for living as our truest and highest self. Ultimately we have to step away from that mindset and stop saying we're sorry for being ourselves. Within this place of being you, there's a balance. The balance is ahimsa, non-harming. This concept returns within the broader sense of daily life. It's crucial not to throw your feelings to the wind or become smaller just because someone can't handle your light. Your highest self exudes authenticity, awareness, and confidence. Within your highest self, you are committing to no longer being a people pleaser.

One of the main characteristics of a people pleaser is saying I'm sorry and apologizing constantly, even when something is not yours to own. It floats along the same shores of being likable, easygoing, and what we have capitalized on as being drama free. Hopefully these practices have opened you up enough to see that it's better to address problems, instead of using your energy to avoid discomfort. When you "please" and "sorry" your way through an issue, it only creates personal stress, and more than likely, the problem will rise again. In the moment it feels safe to make others happy and give the impression of saving the day. In reality, there's nothing more powerful and divinely heart-centered than saying, "No,

I'm done with being a people-pleaser. I'm no longer sorry for being and taking care of me."

Conceptually it's easy to say, yet your inner dialogue is not so convinced. Like yoga and meditation, elevating out of people-pleaser mode takes practice. You have to start with small situations and work your way into the huge conversations. In every instance, you have to clearly state what you are feeling without downplaying your emotions. I find the best way to start is with people you don't know, so there's zero emotional attachment. For example, if you are in a ride and the driver stops to drop you at the corner of your street, but you prefer to be delivered to your address, don't be afraid to push back. More times than not, asserting yourself will garner a positive response. Keep in mind, though, that some people will have a negative response. But really, that's not your fault if you operated from a place of authenticity and kindness. Part of this is not taking ownership of someone else's "bad day." This approach is not harsh or what some call being unyogic-like. It's being honest. Mini practices will give you the strength to tackle the hard interactions.

I want you to visualize your most divine self. What is your posture? What are your eyes doing? What is the quality of your breath? As you may know, your body language carries far more weight than the words you speak. Even if the butterflies are spinning, the way you carry yourself is far more convincing when it comes to holding your ground. Showing personal conviction and not cowering is about making eye contact and being okay with taking up space with your physical body. But in the state of being authentically you, it's also important to be connected to the flow of your breath and listen fully. As you merge the full range of body language with your words, the message will be received more fully, even if the other person doesn't like what you are delivering. Don't be afraid; it all comes back to authenticity, awareness, and confidence.

DIVINE IN LOVE

I haven't yet touched on the topic of intimate relationships in the age of texting and online dating. I felt it was important to discuss it in this section because by now you are maybe experiencing pushback in a current relationship, or wondering how much of yourself you should expose in a new relationship, or how to fully be yourself when you are single and ready to mingle.

Your age, gender, or sexual orientation has nothing to do with being divinely you while falling in love. We've all turned down the light of our soul in order to find love. This has nothing to do with anyone else. It's not the person you are married to, dating, or considering dating. Pretending to be their version of you, circles back to you. What you are experiencing in a relationship is all you. There are definitely narcissists and energy vampires floating in the dating pool, but when you elevate into your fullness, they see the light and run. They exit and refrain from entering your life because relationships are a reflection of what is happening inside you.

It's easy to minimize a wonky character defect or dysfunctional behavior because you are suppressing it in yourself or you haven't addressed that shadow. You may not see it immediately, but after a few disagreements and disappointments, it rises to the top. Also it may not appear in the same form as your shadow but instead surfaces as a different unhealthy quality.

One of my clients dated a guy for over two years. During their time together she struggled with a variety of things, but they all related to communication and showing up as a partner. He viewed her as selfish and unable to nurture him, complained that she was devoted to everyone else, and repeatedly told her she would miss him when he was gone. As she evaluated her needs in the relationship, reconnected to her inner voice, committed to a personal practice based on self-love, and spoke honestly about how she felt, the guy dismissed himself from the relationship via text. In the end, it all came down to her settling into old patterns, compromising her values, and making every attempt to make him happy. Taking on the "you complete me" mentality never works. If you aren't happy and working on you, you are bound to attract a jealous, controlling, and even manipulative partner.

So what do you do? Well, you definitely have to do the inner work. This doesn't mean your house is forever clean and free of issues. It means you have to know your issues, actively work on them, and be honest about who you are. You also can't compromise. Take your time in the dating process. If a red flag surfaces or you experience a quality that impacts your personal values, say goodbye without apologizing. If you are showing up as you and not hiding your love of self, the partner you are with will do the same. Let go of the opposites attract idea and welcome a relationship centered in personal wholeness. Even if you are married, you want a partner that radiates the same life force.

MEDITATION TO PREVENT FREAKING OUT

When you are in the process of delivering uncomfortable news, speaking to a group of people, or even taking the initial steps of living fully as yourself, fear creeps in. Honestly, fear is always going to be there, but I have another tool in the toolbox. The following meditation is designed to alter your overall energy of anxiety and irritation or assist you in managing a neurotic state. It enhances your ability to breathe through both nostrils and to balance fire (*agni*) and coolness (*sitali*) in the body and mind.

HOW TO PRACTICE   Sit in a comfortable cross-legged position with a straight spine, a gentle neck lock, and relaxed shoulders. Interlace your fingers with your right thumb on top. Place your hands on your diaphragm. Close your eyes and breathe while focusing your attention on the tip of your nose. Observe which nostril you are mainly breathing from. If you notice the breathing coming from the left nostril, consciously shift it to the right, and vice versa. Practice changing the breath back and forth. Start with three minutes and work your way up to thirty-one minutes.

If the breathing pattern doesn't shift immediately do not stress out or try to force it. This meditation comes back to the simplicity of the breath and serves as a practice to keep calm and focused.

UNAPOLOGETIC DATING TIPS

The following is a list of tips for dating unapologetically.

- **Be you.** Show up as your highest self and don't switch gears when you start dating. Dialing it back and not being who you are will never work. Lead with confidence, let your radiance shine, and speak up when something is uncomfortable or doesn't sit well with your core values. In addition, it's important to be independent and maintain a vibrant life outside of your partner. The person meant for you will always understand, appreciate, and encourage your glow.

- **Communicate.** Texting is a new form of communication. It is not the way we as humans form and cultivate quality relationships. Even if you meet someone online, get off the app and meet in person. Don't extend the time before you meet. I'm old school; if a potential partner asks you out via text, don't be afraid to respond with, "Hey, let's jump on the phone to set a time and place." This is about being clear in the beginning about what form of communication you value. As a result, when you need to chat about something serious, it will be easier to discuss face-to-face, and you will feel comfortable connecting with truth and vulnerability.

Another word on texting: Regardless of one's job, it should never take hours or days to respond to a text. If someone isn't responding or the conversation is a one-way thread, put down the phone and swim away. Also beware of late-night-only texts, drunk texts, and the flood of texts that never lead to meeting in person. Again, texting is a new form for communication, but it is not a substitute for cultivating and maintaining a healthy relationship.

- **Be aware of your energetic investment**. Energetic investment goes both ways. If you are single, be aware of the amount of time you are investing in someone and make sure they're investing equally in you. In the busyness of life, there are times when you have more time than the person you are connecting with. But if your partner only wants to watch Netflix and chill, or their version of a date is hanging with family and friends, exit stage right. Be clear about your standards and relationship needs. Remain conscious of your energetic investment, and remain true to what you personally deserve.

- **Have fun**. Dating is more than getting boo'd up after the first date. Dating is about determining your likes, dislikes, needs, and overall desires. With all of the work you've done so far, you aren't thirsty. You are a magnificent catch, so go out and swim in the sea with other great catches. Along the way, you will float past someone and there will be an organic spark. Even in that moment, drop in and see how it evolves.

Now that you have a few basic dating tips, I want you to get clear about what you desire in a partner. Being a divine human with a captivating aura, it's only natural that people will gravitate to you. When it comes to intimate relationships, I've learned from my own life and the lives of friends and clients that it's crucial to know what you want and to make a list of those characteristics in the same way you contemplated and created a list for your deepest passions; you can't leave this love thing to chance. I don't care what some of those dating gurus say online, you can't make someone fall in love with you, and you aren't the type to play mind games.

DIVINE LOVER MEDITATION AND LIST

Through this next exercise, I want you to create a list of characteristics, traits, energetic qualities, feelings, and anything else you need your partner to have when it comes to being your divine lover.

HOW TO PRACTICE Come onto your back, close your eyes, and take about ten to fifteen breaths through your nose. While taking these breaths, allow your entire body to slowly relax from your feet to the crown of your head. Imagine yourself in your favorite place in world. You are alone, and you are soaking up the complete experience. Maybe you are walking, dancing, or being present in stillness. Your eyes and heart are breathing in each moment filled with delight, joy, and pure happiness. There's so much glee that you could stay there forever. After a few minutes, out of the corner of your eye you see your lover walking toward you. Seeing this person reminds you how wonderful it is to enjoy this moment with a partner that loves, honors, and respects all of who you are. The two of you hold hands and begin to experience your blissful moment together as divine equals. Stay here for as long as you wish. When you are ready to come out, gently move your body and slowly open your eyes.

Open your journal and begin to make your list of divine lover qualities. Don't second-guess yourself and don't settle. The words you are writing reflect your deepest yearning to move in tandem with someone just as Spiritually Fly as you. Put it all down, review it periodically, and add to the list when you need to.

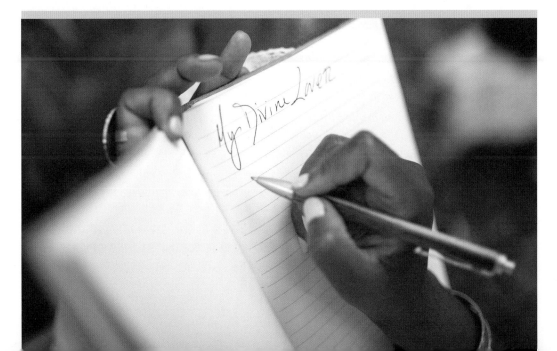

DIVINE MOTHER OF SWEETNESS

The practices shared in this book are tools for cultivating inner strength, cleansing the body, purifying the soul, and building a foundation for personal evolution. Over the past nine years, I've completely reshaped my connection to self, crafted a life methodology based solely on energy and experience, and realigned the way I live in the world. Along with ancient teachings and self-study, I tested, recorded, and cataloged all of my personal and teaching practices. As you've probably noticed, I've found African teachings extremely valuable. Although they are not connected to what many modern yogis consider yoga, I find these teachings to be influential and heavily connected to my Spiritually Fly life. I love these teachings because they draw upon my own divine qualities and my African roots. I've merged them throughout the book, and it felt extremely appropriate to include one more in the final chapter.

It was the summer of 2004, and I jumped on a New York City subway and a made a trip to Brooklyn with a boyfriend who studied Afro-Brazilian culture. As we entered a fourth-floor walk-up, I felt the supernatural channels of life and death floating around my body. I'd always been sensitive to others' energy, but there was something familiar and comfortable in the pathways. My boyfriend was going to speak with a Candomblé priestess, and I had no idea what that really meant. I was definitely intrigued, and I decided it was worth a day into the unknown.

While gazing upon the spiritual symbols on the walls and altar, I felt a calmness. It reminded me of when I walked into the hospital room after my brother died. I felt united with life and death and centered in love. Thoughts from the day lingered in my mind later on, but for the life of me I couldn't remember the name of the priestess. I did, however, remember her repeating the word Oxúm over and over while she touched my hand. The priestess only spoke in Portuguese, so upon returning to our apartment in Harlem, my boyfriend summarized the bulk of the visit for me. The major piece was that the goddess Oxúm lived within me, and the priestess saw it the moment I walked in. As years passed, I began to learn more about African religions, and Yoruba spiritual traditions specifically. Around 2014, I began to share some the philosophy with my yoga classes and workshops.

Candomblé is a religion found primarily in Brazil that is heavily influenced by the African beliefs and traditions of the Yoruba, Bantu, and Fon peoples. During the slave trade, between the sixteenth and nineteenth centuries,

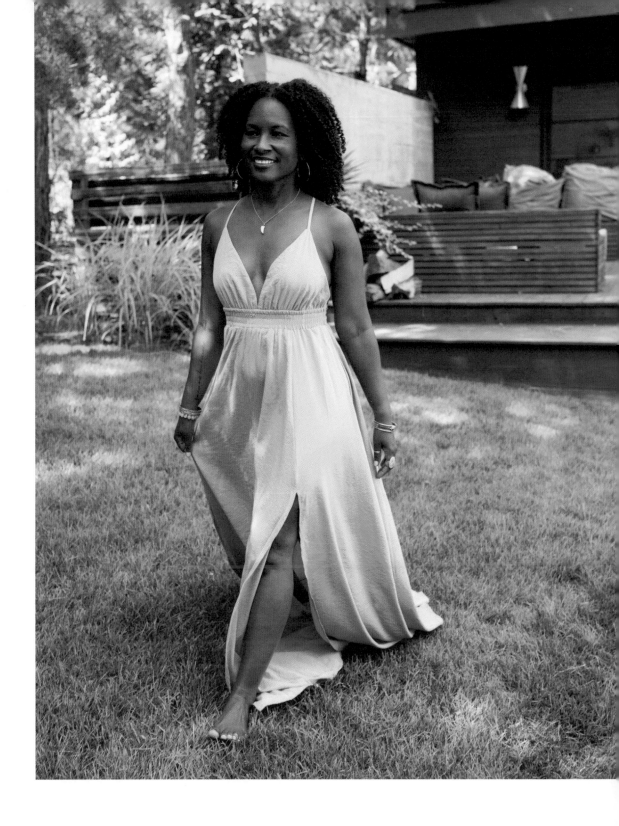

Africans who were brought to Brazil merged the spiritual traditions of their homeland with a few aspects of Catholicism. Out of this beautiful creation came Candomblé.

Candomblé means "dance in honor of the gods." Within the teachings there is one powerful god called Oludumaré, who is supported by other gods and goddesses called Orixás, who are divine forces of nature much like the assortment of gods and goddesses within the Hindu philosophy. It is believed that each person has their own Orixá resting within them that acts as a protector and is formed with you. The goddess Oxúm (also spelled Oshun) is often characterized as the Orixá of love, beauty, sensuality, and femininity; however, her powers reach further into the vast realms of womanhood (from young girl to wise elder). In Haiti she is referred to as Erzulie or Ezili. Within the *patakís* (sacred teachings left by our ancestors), Oxúm was created by Oludumaré to add sweetness and love to the earth. Her divine love is manifested in warmth, compassion, fertility, prosperity, good cheer, and ultimate joy, and flows along all fresh waters around the world. Within the stories, the human race would not exist if Oxúm were not sent to bring sweet life to us mortals. For me, this spiritual practice cultivates steadiness and fluidity because it blends beautiful traditions from Africa and the Americas even though it evolves from slavery. I view Candomblé as a perfect balance of ancient teachings that supports our ability to live within our current human existence.

During the years of my own healing, I began to see the qualities of Oxúm reflected in the mirror she carries. In Western culture, carrying a mirror may be seen as vain, but for Oxúm, the mirror represents our divine self-image. Through breath, movement, chanting, and pure spiritual devotion, I began to see the qualities of compassion, creativity, vitality, grace, abundance, beauty, sensuality, femininity, and of course, love emanate from my heart. Most of all, my healing practices knocked down the walls and cleared a path so I could see myself as a mother who nourishes and supports humanity through my dharma. This spiritual awakening enabled me to live unapologetically as myself in all areas of my life.

During workshops and special events, I love incorporating Oxúm into the flow of the moment. Her mirror becomes a form of introspective meditation, a peacock feather appears on the altar, the color yellow surfaces as flowers or clothing, gold shines in my own jewelry, and sweetness pours like honey through music and the tone of my voice.

MOTHER OF SWEETNESS MEDITATION

This meditation merged with sound is designed to help you drop into the arms of Mother Oxúm and feel held by her love. Many musical artists have been inspired by her blessings, and as a result they crafted many songs in honor of her beauty. The one I love most is the Oshun (Oxúm) Chant by the Women of the Calabash (see below). Their voices echo along the curves of your body and pulsate like heaven in the soul.

OSHUN CHANT

Ide were were nita Oshun
Ide were were, Ide were
    were nita Oshun
Ide were were nita ya,
    Ocha kiniba nita Oshun
Cheké, Cheké, Cheké nita
    ya, Ide were were

Before you start, locate this version online then play it while enjoying the following moving meditation. If your spirit prompts you, hit repeat and continue to move.

HOW TO PRACTICE   Stand with your feet about six to eight inches apart. Begin to play the track. Close your eyes for five to seven breaths and feel the rhythm and vibrations. Then begin to intuitively move your body. This can be done with your eyes open or closed. The idea is to be with the energy of Oxúm and dance in celebration of your divinity. When you are ready to stop, return to the starting position. Close your eyes, breathe for ten to twenty breaths, and feel Oxúm holding you lovingly in her sweetness.

Being your divine self without apologizing is about gathering all of the lessons you've learned on the mat, in meditation, and throughout the ups and downs of life and using them to craft the life you desire. To further support you on this spiritual journey, I've expanded this final chapter to include three yin yoga postures to support you when life is spinning, a kundalini kriya to nourish your beautiful soul, and three kundalini meditations to keep you elevated. All of these cultivate mindfulness, awareness, strength, and divine love.

yoga practice
your true divine self

Yin yoga is a lovely and delicious meditative practice that helps us energetically heal through stillness in the yoga postures. It calms the mind while targeting the connective tissues between the muscles and fascia. The following three yin yoga poses are designed to cultivate a sweet balance between body and soul. Before moving into the practice, you may want to grab a pillow or blanket as a support. Allow yourself to surrender and just breathe.

mantra

I live my divine life without apologizing.

EXTENDED CHILD'S POSE (*UTTHITA BALASANA*)   All you need to do in this pose is let go and rest. The gentle elongation of the spine relieves tension in the back while also providing a great stretch. Because it falls in the category of being a less active posture, you can easily support your head and torso on a pillow or blanket, which helps to relieve any discomfort you may experience in the neck. It also stretches your ankles, hips, and thighs. Because it is a forward fold, it also massages the abdominal organs. Therapeutically, it's great for relieving mental and emotional fatigue and stress and for cooling for menopause.

HOW TO PRACTICE   Come onto all fours. Open your knees wider than your hips and bring your big toes together to touch. Breathe in and as you exhale, slowly draw your hips toward your feet and rest your buttocks on your heels. You are going to stay here for several minutes, so if it's uncomfortable, place a pillow or rolled blanket under your chest. You can also slide the blanket between your heels and hips. Your arms may remain slightly extended and relaxed. Take slow, easy breaths and stay in the posture for three to six minutes. Release from the posture very slowly by returning to your hands and knees. Have a seat and gently shake your legs out.

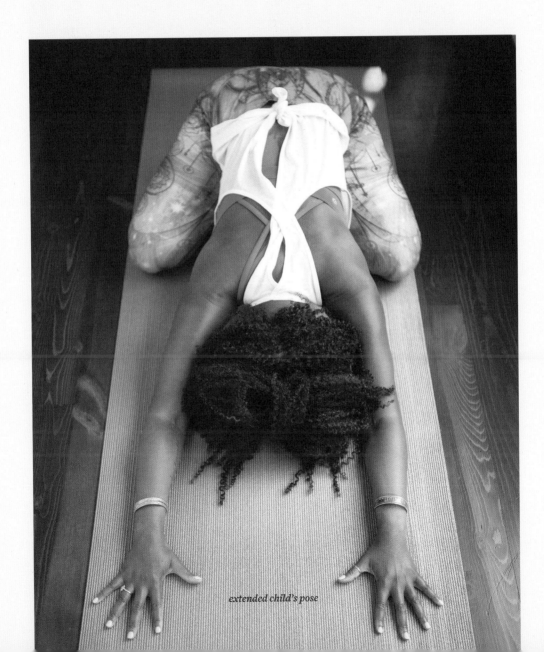

extended child's pose

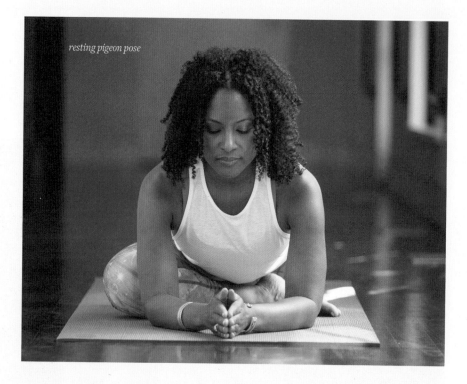

resting pigeon pose

RESTING PIGEON POSE (*EKA PADA RAJAKAPOTASANA*)   This is one of the yummiest and most dreaded poses in hatha yoga. Because it works on stretching and increasing the mobility in the hips, many people love it and others absolutely hate it. Energetically it stimulates the second chakra and supports the release of emotions while improving fluidity, and it is great at igniting those hips for sexual intimacy. Because this is the resting variation, the pose enables you to fold forward. The folding action calms the mind and softens the heart, and like Child's Pose, it massages the abdominal organs. I also find the overall essence, mental and physical, makes it a beautiful prep pose for long meditations.

HOW TO PRACTICE   From all fours, bring your right knee forward toward your right wrist or slightly behind it. At this point you may want to place a blanket or pillow under your right hip. The key is to see how flexible you are and judge whether you can release into the pose without support. Because most of us have tight hips, the right ankle will likely land closer to the left hip than the left wrist.

Take a deep inhale, and on the exhale walk your hands forward and release your chest, head, and arms past your right leg. Your left leg remains extended behind you with the top of your foot on the mat. Hold the posture for two to four minutes. Breathe slowly and deeply. You can also place a pillow under your forehead. To come out, inhale and walk your hands back until they are under the shoulders. Release onto your right hip and swing your left leg forward. Give your legs a little shake, return to all fours, and do the same on the left side.

RECLINED SPINAL TWIST (*SUPTA MATSYENDRASANA*)   There's no better way to end the set of hatha postures shared in this book than with Reclined Spinal Twist. Like the other postures in this set, it provides a soothing yet extremely effective massage for the abdominal muscles while also strengthening them. As it tones the waistline, it also provides a subtle detox by stimulating the digestive system. With the arms open in a T-shape, it stretches the shoulders, expands the chest, and gets into the upper back. It also stretches down the muscles of the spine to the glutes and aligns the spine. As an added plus, it calms the mind and literally squeezes out stress.

HOW TO PRACTICE   Lie on your back with your legs extended. Inhale and draw your left knee into your chest. Shift your hips slightly to the left. On the exhale, release your knee to the right side of your body, resting your right hand on the outside of your left knee. Allow your left arm to open to the left in line with your left shoulder. You can remain here or open your right arm in line with your right shoulder. Both palms are facing up. As you hold the pose, keep your left knee drawn in near your chest so the lower back remains open and stretched. You have the option of turning the head to the left or keeping it straight. Let gravity take over and hold the posture for one to two minutes while breathing gently through the nose. Slowly return to center and extend the left leg along the floor. Take two to five breaths and repeat on the other side. For added comfort or support, you can place a blanket or pillow under your knee, or you can do the twist with both knees bent.

KUNDALINI KRIYA: KEEPING THE BODY BEAUTIFUL

This kriya balances the prana *vayu* energy (the inward and upward flow of air) and *apana vayu* energy (the air that moves down and out) within the body, which is great for digestion. As it balances the natural flow of vital energy, it will cleanse and neutralize the entire system.

HOW TO PRACTICE   Sit in a comfortable cross-legged position with your spine straight. Place your hands on your knees and take long, deep breaths through the nose. Do this for three minutes. At the last inhale, hold the breath for a few seconds, then exhale slowly and move on to the following poses.

FROG POSE   Stand with your toes turned out and your heels slightly touching. Fold forward and bend your knees to squat on the balls of your feet, with your knees spread apart. Make sure your heels are touching and raised off the floor. Place the tips of your fingers a few inches in front of your feet on the floor and gaze forward. As you inhale, raise your hips and straighten your legs, keeping the heels up and fingers touching the ground. Exhale and bend the knees (returning to the squat) with your face forward. Repeat this ten times. On the tenth round, remain in the squat and take three long, deep breaths. On the third breath, exhale fully and hold the breath for ten to twenty seconds while engaging the root lock. Repeat the Frog Pose movement twenty-six more times. On the last one, remain in the squat and take three deep breaths, hold the third breath, and engage the root lock. Lower your heels and slowly lift your upper body. Pause for a few breaths while standing and notice the sensations.

Note: This can be a very intense movement. If your lower back or hamstrings are tight, you can modify the pose by lowering your heels when you straighten your legs. Also, only bend your knees as much as is comfortable and move at your own pace.

FRONT STRETCH   Sit on the floor and extend your legs straight out in front of you. Fold forward and grab your big toes with your index and middle fingers and thumbs. On the inhale, lengthen your spine by reaching your chest forward. Exhale and fold gently from the navel center, allowing your chest to release toward your thighs. Avoid forcefully reaching with your head and simply let it soften. Breathe through your nose and hold the pose for three minutes. At the end, inhale, hold the breath for a few seconds, then exhale slowly. Gently release on your back for a three-minute Corpse Pose.

This kriya can be followed by any of the following meditations.

Kundalini Meditations

The following meditations serve as practices to support your continued spiritual work, elevate you when needed, and aid you in maintaining inner balance.

MEDITATION FOR ABSOLUTELY POWERFUL ENERGY The power of *Ong* vibrates through the entire body via the sushumna nadi. It elevates the consciousness, balances the brain, and energizes all aspects of your being.

HOW TO PRACTICE Sit in a comfortable cross-legged position and engage a neck lock with the spine straight. Interlace your fingers, then extend your ring fingers and bring them to touch at a 60-degree angle. Place your right thumb over your left thumb and hold your hands a few inches from your diaphragm. Close your eyes. Inhale fully and powerfully chant *Ong* in a continuous vibration for at least five times.

MEDITATION TO TOTALLY RECHARGE YOU This meditation is perfect for easing depression, handling life's shifts and changes, and connecting you to the depth of the breath.

HOW TO PRACTICE Sit in a comfortable cross-legged position and engage a neck lock with the spine straight. Lift your arms in front of your chest so they are parallel to the floor. With straight arms, wrap your left fingers around your right fist. Your thumbs extend up and touch on the sides while your palms touch at the base. Focus your eyes on your thumbs. Inhale for five seconds, then exhale for five seconds and suspend the breath out for fifteen seconds. Do this for three to five minutes and slowly work your way up to eleven minutes. Soon you will have the capacity to suspend the breath for a full minute.

MEDITATION TO BRIGHTEN YOUR RADIANCE This meditation is great for projecting out your inner radiance. It's like your inner glow stick shines.

HOW TO PRACTICE Sit in a comfortable cross-legged position with a straight spine. Bring your hands to about twelve inches from your ears with your palms facing forward and your elbows bent. Bring your hands into gyan mudra with your thumbs and index fingers together and the other fingers extended to the sky. Focus your gaze on the tip of your nose. Create an O shape with your mouth and breathe long and deep through the mouth for twenty-one minutes. If this is too long a time for you at first, start out with three minutes and slowly build up. At the end, inhale fully and hold the breath for twenty seconds, then exhale slowly.

Reaching the moment when you have pulled back the layers of your existence and finally revealed ALL that you are can be really scary. This is the moment where you pause, collect your thoughts, ground down, and breathe into your Flyness. When you feel a little shaky or your palms start to sweat, remember all the work you've done to live unapologetically. Don't cast darkness over your own shine, don't make excuses for why you say no, and definitely don't explain your YES to living your life. I encourage you to remember the magnitude of your divinity. For the spirits of all the Orixás, heaven and earth, and mystics and ancestors are part of a never-ending wellspring within you. So know you will rise and you will fall, but you will always continue to grow. Be in the movement of navigating the layers of relationships with friends, family, romantic partners, and the self, but always be in the place of honoring the source of your worth. I'll tell you what one of my elders told me: "Grab a bigger cup, because you have so much more of your amazing life to drink."